How to Become a Counselling Psychologist

Counselling psychologists can play a fundamental and inspiring role in people's lives. Their aim is to address a range of psychological and emotional issues, helping people to live more skilful, effective, and meaningful lives. But how do you qualify, and what is being a counselling psychologist really like?

How to Become a Counselling Psychologist is the first book to provide a clear, practical guide to the pathway to qualifying as a counselling psychologist. Written by an experienced practitioner, and incorporating testimonials from trainees, trainers, and qualified counselling psychologists, it explains every step of the journey, including advice on choosing a suitable degree course, making the most of a training placement, preparing for the job interview, and negotiating the challenges of making the transition from training to qualification.

Written for anyone from current students to those interested in a change of career, *How to Become a Counselling Psychologist* is an indispensable guide for anyone interested in this rich and varied branch of psychology.

Dr Elaine Kasket, C.Psychol. is an HCPC-Registered Counselling Psychologist and Principal Lecturer in Counselling Psychology at Regent's University, London, UK, where she also heads the professional doctorate. She is well-acquainted with the "portfolio" professional identity that is familiar to so many counselling psychologists, having worked as a trainer, practitioner, supervisor, researcher, and writer within the field.

GW00499000

How to Become a Practitioner Psychologist

Series Editor: David Murphy, University of Oxford

David Murphy, FBPsS is Co-Director of the Oxford Institute of Clinical Psychology Training and a fellow of Harris Manchester College, University of Oxford. He is Past Chair of the Professional Practice Board of the British Psychological Society and has also been Director of the BPS Division of Clinical Psychology – Professional Standards Unit.

How to Become a Counselling Psychologist
Elaine Kasket

How to Become a Sport and Exercise Psychologist
Martin Eubank and David Tod

How to Become a Counselling Psychologist

Elaine Kasket

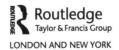

Routledge
Taylor & Francis Group

LONDON AND NEW YORK

First published 2017
by Routledge
2 Park Square, Milton Park, Abingdon, Oxon OX14 4RN

and by Routledge
711 Third Avenue, New York, NY 10017

Routledge is an imprint of the Taylor & Francis Group, an informa business

British Library Cataloguing in Publication Data
A catalogue record for this book is available from the British Library

Library of Congress Cataloging in Publication Data
A catalog record for this book has been requested

ISBN: 978-1-138-94821-1 (hbk)
ISBN: 978-1-138-94824-2 (pbk)
ISBN: 978-1-315-66967-0 (ebk)

Typeset in Galliard
by Swales & Willis, Exeter, Devon, UK

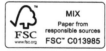

MIX
Paper from
responsible sources
FSC
www.fsc.org   FSC™ C013985

Printed in the United Kingdom
by Henry Ling Limited

This book is dedicated to all of the hard-working trainee and qualified counselling psychologists who have shared their experiences with me in service of helping, inspiring and guiding future generations of professionals. I am terrifically pleased to have them as my colleagues.

I also dedicate it to Zoe, the star at the centre of my orbit, who twinkles with a lovely and inspiring light.

Contents

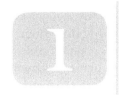

Introduction

David Murphy – Series
Editor

Welcome!

First, I would like to welcome you to this book, which is one of a series of seven titles, each of which focuses on a different type of practitioner psychologist registered as a professional in the UK. One of the things that has always appealed to me about psychology is its incredible diversity; even within my own primary field of clinical psychology there is a huge range of client groups and ways of working. The books in this series are all written by practitioner psychologists who are not only experts in, but hugely enthusiastic about, each of their areas of practice. This series presents a fascinating insight into the nature of each domain and the range of activities and approaches within it, and also the fantastic variety there is across the different areas of practice. However, we have also made sure that we have answered the practical questions you may have such as "How long does it take to train?", "What do I need to do to get on a training course?" and "How secure will my income be at the end of it all?" We very much hope that this book will be interesting and answer all your questions (even ones you didn't know you had!) and further information and resources are available on our series website (www.routledge.com/cw/howto becomeapractitionerpsychologist).

Psychology as a profession

Psychology is still a relatively young profession compared to many long-established professions such as law, medicine, accounting, etc., however it has grown incredibly rapidly over the last few decades. One

1

of the first people to use the title "Psychologist" in a professional context was Lightner Witmer who established what is widely recognised as the world's first psychology clinic in 1896 in Pennsylvania. Witmer came to study psychology after a degree in Economics and postgraduate studies in political science and then working for a time as a school teacher. He went on to study experimental psychology at the University of Pennsylvania and then at a famous laboratory in Germany. Witmer went on to pioneer the application of experimental psychology ideas to the treatment of children with specific learning and speech difficulties.

At the beginning of the twentieth century, these early psychologists saw great possibilities in applying psychological concepts to help people achieve their potential. However, even they could scarcely imagine the scale and range of applications of psychology that would exist by the beginning of the twenty-first century. Psychologists now have well-established roles in schools, mental and physical health services, prisons, police and security services, multi-national companies, sport training centres; essentially almost anywhere where there is a focus on understanding and changing human behaviour, which is, of course, pretty much everywhere!

This book is, along with the other six titles in the series, intended to provide people who are at the beginning of their careers, or those who are thinking about making a change, an insight into the different areas of professional psychology. We hope that you will not only gain an overview of what the specific domain of psychology entails, but also a sense of what it is like to work as a practitioner on a day-to-day basis. We also aim to explain how to become qualified to practice in the area of professional psychology, right from school until being fully qualified. Furthermore, we hope to provide an idea of how careers in the different areas of psychology can develop over time and how the profession of psychology might change as it continues to develop in the future.

Studying psychology at school or college

One thing that many people love about psychology is just how broad it is. As an academic discipline it encompasses physiological workings of the brain and the nervous system, how we perceive sounds and language, how we make decisions and the treatment of mental health problems, to name just a few areas. In recent years psychology has become the second most popular degree subject at UK universities – indeed a total of 72,000 students were studying, either full-time or part-time, for a first degree in psychology in the academic year 2014–15.

Psychology has become not only a popular A-level choice but also increasingly an option at GCSE level. It is now possible, therefore, to take the first step on a career journey in psychology at an early age, and, if you are considering A-levels or GCSE subjects, we would certainly encourage you to look at psychology options if they are offered at your school. However, it is by no means required to have studied psychology at GCSE or A-level to follow a career in psychology. If you have already taken other subjects, or psychology isn't offered at your school, or you have decided to go for other subjects, this won't stop you going on to become a psychologist, if you decide that this is what you would like to do. Furthermore, contrary to some myths, psychology is considered a valid A-level choice for many other degrees apart from psychology; indeed it is listed as a "preferred subject" by University College London in their general list of A-level subject choices: see http://www.ucl.ac.uk/prospective-students/undergraduate/application/requirements/preferred-a-level-subjects

The only GCSE subjects that are specifically required by UK universities to study psychology are maths and English. A-level psychology is usually listed as a "preferred" subject but is currently not required by any UK university for entry to a psychology course, and there is no indication that this will change. Therefore, overall our advice would be that psychology is an interesting subject choice which can provide a good foundation for further study in psychology, or other subjects. However, psychology at A-level is by no means essential for a career as a psychologist, so we recommend basing the decision on what your strengths and interests are and also what subjects are required for any other degree options you want to keep open to you.

Studying psychology at university

The first compulsory step on the road to a psychology career is attaining "Graduate Basis for Chartered Membership" of the British Psychological Society, commonly known as "GBC" (in the past this was called "Graduate Basis for Registration" or "GBR" for short). You will see this referred to a number of times in this book and the other titles in the series. The British Psychological Society (BPS) is the professional body and learned society for psychology in the United Kingdom. It was established in 1901 to promote both academic and applied psychology and currently has over 50,000 members, making it one of the largest psychological societies in the world. There are two possible routes to attaining Graduate Basis for Chartered Membership of the British Psychological Society on the basis of UK qualifications.

The most common route is to complete an undergraduate degree in psychology that is accredited by the BPS; a lower second class degree classification or above is required. This doesn't need to be a single honours degree in psychology; it can be a joint degree with another subject. However, in order to be accredited it has to cover a core curriculum that is specified by the BPS, and the provision must meet certain standards. At the time of writing there are over 950 BPS-accredited courses offered at over 125 different higher education institutions within the UK. Many of these courses are general psychology degrees; however, some focus more on specific domains such as forensic psychobiology, health psychology, abnormal psychology, sport psychology, business psychology, and so forth. Many are offered as psychology combined with another subject, and the array of possible options is extensive, including business, English literature, education, maths, history, philosophy, physics, zoology, and criminology, to name but a few. This range of choice could be a little bit overwhelming, but it is important to bear in mind that virtually all psychology degrees do offer a significant choice of options within them, so two students doing the same generic psychology degree at the same institution may actually take quite a different mix of courses, albeit still with the same core psychology components. Moreover, it is also important to remember that even if the title of a degree appears very specific, the course will still cover the same core psychology content.

For a career in professional psychology, the most important issue is attaining GBC. The subtle differences in the individual course content are far less important. Our advice would be to consider all the factors that are important to you about the choice of university and the psychology course rather than getting too focused on the specific content of a course. You may wish to do a degree that allows you to specialise in the area of psychology that you are particularly interested in, and of course that's fine. However, in reality, all postgraduate professional training courses need to cater for people with a range of different psychology backgrounds, so whilst having completed specialised options at undergraduate level might provide a good foundation to build on, it is very unlikely to mean that you can jump ahead of those who didn't do those options at undergraduate level.

My own experience was that I did a joint degree with psychology and zoology (I wasn't really sure what psychology was when I was choosing, so I hedged my bets!). Fairly early on I became interested in clinical psychology but I still got a great deal out of studying other subjects that weren't anything to do with clinical psychology, including many of the zoology subjects. In my final year, I did an option in vertebrate paleontology (better known as the study of dinosaurs!), mainly because it sounded interesting. In fact, it turned out to be one of the most stimulating and useful courses I have ever studied, and the lecturer was one of the best teachers I have ever come across. I learned how to interpret inconclusive evidence by using careful observation and deduction rather than jumping to conclusions, and that generic skill has been very useful through my clinical psychology career. So my personal advice would be not to feel under any pressure to specialise in a particular branch of psychology too soon. I suggest you choose degree options because they are stimulating and well taught, *not* because you think they will look good on your CV. In reality, if you are applying for professional psychology training courses, what will stand out more on your CV will be really good grades which come from being really engaged and developing a thorough understanding of the areas you are studying.

Some psychology programmes offer a "professional placement year" within the degree. Such courses are often marketed on the basis that graduates have a higher employment rate on graduation. It is important to bear in mind, however, that you will also be graduating a year later than people on a three-year course, and during the placement year most people will be receiving little or no pay and still paying fees (albeit at a reduced rate) to the university. My own personal opinion is that degrees with professional placements don't necessarily offer an advantage overall. On the one hand, if a course does offer well-established placement opportunities, this can make it easier to get that first step on the ladder; however, there are many opportunities for getting postgraduate experience relevant to professional psychology, some of which are voluntary but many of which are paid.

The other main route to GBC is designed for people who have done first degrees in subjects other than psychology, and enables them to attain GBC by doing a conversion course. At the time of writing there were 67 BPS accredited conversion courses in the UK. Most of these lead to an MSc, although some lead to a graduate diploma; some are general in their content and are titled simply "Psychology" or "Applied psychology", whereas others are more focused on specific areas like child development, mental health or even fashion. However, if they are BPS accredited all of these courses will still cover the core psychology curriculum, regardless of their title.

Since the core components are common between all BPS-accredited degree programmes, you certainly will not be committing yourself irrevocably to any one area of professional psychology through your choice of psychology undergraduate or postgraduate conversion course. In the clinical psychology programme that I run, we take people who have a range of different experiences at undergraduate level, and some who did different degrees altogether. Of course, when you come to postgraduate qualifications, you do have to make more fundamental choices about the area of psychology you wish to focus on.

The different areas of psychology practice

The authors of each of the seven books in the series are, as you would expect, experts in, and enthusiastic about, their own area of psychology practice, and the rest of this book will focus pretty much exclusively on this specific area. Our aim across the series is to provide information about what each domain is about, what it is like to work in this area on a day-to-day basis, and what the route to becoming qualified is like. What we have not done, and indeed could not do, is say which one of the domains is "best" for you. The answer is that there is no one "best" type of psychologist. Instead, we hope you will be able to find the area of practice that seems to fit your own interests and strengths best. This can be difficult, and we would encourage you to keep an open mind for as long as you can; you might be surprised to find that an area you hadn't really thought much about seems to be a good fit.

Once you have identified an area of practice that seems to fit you best, we would certainly recommend that you try and meet people who work in that area and talk to them personally. Even after you have embarked on postgraduate training in a particular field, don't feel it is too late to explore other areas. Indeed, there are areas of overlap between the different domains, and psychologists with different training backgrounds might well end up working in a similar area. For instance clinical and counselling psychologists often work together in psychological therapy services in the NHS, whereas health psychologists and occupational psychologists might work alongside each other in implementing employee health programmes.

My own journey in professional psychology started with my degree in psychology and zoology, as mentioned earlier, and led onto postgraduate training in clinical psychology and then working in the National Health Service. However, my journey also included going on to be registered as a health psychologist and a clinical neuropsychologist, and I went on to do management training and became a senior manager in the NHS before moving into clinical psychology training and research in leadership development. Over the years, I have worked alongside colleagues from all of the domains at various times, particularly through roles with the British Psychological Society. I have been fascinated to learn even more about other domains through editing this series and, of course, as psychology is still such a young and dynamic field, new developments and new fields continue to emerge. I would, therefore, encourage you to think carefully about your career direction, but regardless of whether your psychology "career" lasts just for the duration of this book or the rest of your life, I would encourage you to maintain an open and curious mind. In the words of one of my favourite sayings, "It is better to travel well than to arrive." We hope this book, and the others in the series, will be of help to you, wherever your own unique career journey takes you!

What does a counselling psychologist do?

If you have picked up this book, you must be curious about what a counselling psychologist is, and you may even already be contemplating a career in this profession. You are not alone! Since the British Psychological Society (BPS) launched the Division of Counselling Psychology in 1994, the numbers of trainee and qualified counselling psychologists have grown steadily, showing that a career in counselling psychology is an attractive option for many aspirant practitioner psychologists in the United Kingdom. Statistics kept by the Division chart how interest in the field has risen, with a 25% increase in trainees between 2009 and 2015. Qualified counselling psychologists are now the third most common type of practitioner psychologist in the UK; as of September 2015, there were 2,012 counselling psychologists registered in the country. Increasing awareness of the profession and burgeoning employment opportunities mean that ever-more people are applying for training, either through one of the university-based professional doctorates in counselling psychology scattered around the UK, or via the BPS' Qualification in Counselling Psychology (QCoP).

This title in the *How to Become* series is dedicated to the rich and varied field of counselling psychology, and this chapter will help you think through whether this particular branch of applied psychology might be right for you.

Who is this book for?

I hope this book will be useful to people at many different phases in their lives or careers. You may, for example, be an A-level student, thinking about your options for studying psychology at university and beyond, or a university student studying towards a Bachelor's degree. Although you are probably aware that an undergraduate psychology degree is the necessary first step towards a number of careers, you may be confused about your options. The careers advisors who counsel students about future careers may not be specialist enough to guide you fully, and they may have a less-than-firm grasp on what counselling psychology is, what a counselling psychologist does, and how you can qualify. This book should therefore be a valuable additional source of information for you.

But what if your undergraduate education is far behind you? You may already be a seasoned practitioner in one of the helping professions – a social worker, a counsellor, or a psychotherapist. Perhaps you are even a different type of registered or chartered psychologist, contemplating an additional registration as a counselling psychologist. You may know a bit more about counselling psychology than the average psychology undergraduate, and you may be mulling over the potential professional advantages of expanding your existing qualifications. This book is for you, too, and an even greater percentage of it is relevant, for you have more training considerations and alternatives. First of all, if your undergraduate degree was not in psychology, you will need to investigate a conversion course. You should also peruse any sections that discuss the QCoP, also known as the "independent route". As someone with existing training and experience, you will want to carefully weigh up whether the course route or the QCoP is the better option for you.

The last category of readers for whom this book is relevant consists of people taking a less well-charted path to qualification as a counselling psychologist. If you trained as a psychologist in a country outside the UK, for example, you will have found that organisations in the UK will not immediately recognise or transfer your existing qualifications to enable you to practice as a psychologist here. You may also have found it particularly difficult to get advice and to sift through information on qualifying; members of this particular club often feel unable to navigate and synthesise all of the information from the HCPC, the BPS, the Division of Counselling Psychology, and multiple other sources.

Finally, you may be someone who started your qualification journey on one path, such as the taught-course route, but encountered some bumps in the road. Perhaps the course route was insufficiently flexible for your personal circumstances, or you experienced some other difficulty. Because trainees on courses often have no idea that the QCoP exists as an alternative, they may endure unnecessary anxiety and disappointment and give up on their qualification aspirations prematurely. The reverse scenario may also occur, for the QCoP is an autonomous, self-driven mode of qualifying that may leave some people struggling with a feeling of isolation and wondering whether the course route might be a more workable alternative for them.

Before we go any further, however, we need to tackle the question of what counselling psychology is, for it is a profession that has eluded easy definition and neat summary, and that has long been conflated with allied professions, such as counselling. The fact that this confusion has existed historically, however, should not convey the impression that counselling psychology's identity is diffuse. It has a distinct ethos and a commitment to particular values and perspectives, all of which is covered in the next section.

What is counselling psychology?

While on one hand counselling psychology practitioners are highly diverse, they have a number of things in common, and most of those commonalities exist because of the profession's roots in the humanistic psychology movement that started in the 1960s. A brief review of the core ideas of this movement will help you understand what counselling psychology is all about.

The founders and proponents of the humanistic psychology movement, such as Abraham Maslow and Carl Rogers, thought it unhelpful to try and alleviate human distress through classifying, predicting and trying to influence behaviour. Instead, they emphasised themes of individual freedom, choice, meaning, and responsibility. Arguing that scientific assumptions and psychological theories could actually interfere with understanding each person in their unique experience, humanistic psychologists were instead interested in exploring their clients' worlds, and they felt that this could only be achieved through a particular kind of relationship and interaction. The famous "core conditions" outlined by Carl Rogers describe the kind of therapeutic relationship privileged by humanistic psychologists, one characterised by congruence, genuineness, unconditional positive regard for the client, and *empathy* – a word that refers to the striving to understand what it is like to be the other person.

So, first, true to their humanistic psychology roots, counselling psychologists place a strong emphasis on understanding people as individuals, in their unique contexts. They avoid fitting their clients into predetermined diagnostic, theoretical, or therapeutic molds. Instead, they strive to understand each person as holistically as possible, and they tailor their approach to meet each individual's needs. Because of the need to respond flexibly in this way, counselling psychologists are required to understand and to be proficient in multiple approaches to psychological intervention.

Second, counselling psychologists tend to emphasise wellbeing over psychopathology. Like the founders of humanistic psychology, counselling psychologists believe in the inherent potential for growth in every person, and are interested in using psychological intervention to promote and empower that growth.

Third, counselling psychologists tend to resist a doctor–patient, well-person–sick-person, expert–non-expert dynamic. Although there will always be power differentials within the therapeutic relationship, counselling psychologists strive to level the playing field as much as possible, and they consider the client to be the expert on their own experience. Whether assessing, formulating, or intervening, the counselling psychologist works collaboratively with the client, and both the process and the outcome of psychological therapy is the joint effort of both parties working together.

Fourth, counselling psychologists work towards a particularly high level of self-awareness and refer to themselves as "reflexive practitioners". Part of what this means is that they always try to remain aware of their "own stuff" and how it affects their interactions. Counselling psychologists are required to be highly sensitive to *process*. This includes what is going on within themselves, what is going on between therapist and client, and what may be going on within the client – although the counselling psychologist is always careful about *assuming* that they know what is happening for the client. The development of a high level of reflexivity is a key feature of counselling psychology training and a core competency for the qualified practitioner.

Fifth, and again, honouring the humanistic underpinnings of the profession, counselling psychologists view the therapeutic relationship as a key ingredient of successful psychotherapy. The relationship facilitates trust, understanding, clarity, change, and action. The well-known humanistic-existential psychiatrist and practitioner Irvin Yalom has a mantra: "It's the relationship that heals. It's the relationship that heals. It's the relationship that heals" (Yalom, 2003). The counselling psychologist experiences this as fundamental truth, and nurtures and attends to the therapeutic relationship that is at the heart of the work.

Finally, counselling psychologists *are psychologists* rather than counsellors. An undergraduate degree in psychology is required to enter training, and that degree will be imbued with the more traditional roots of psychological science. Counselling psychologists understand diagnosis and the medical context, and they pay attention to knowledge derived from all kinds of sources – laboratory work, large randomised controlled trials (RCTs), small-scale qualitative studies, case studies, their own and others' practice-based evidence, the individual client in front of them, and the dynamics of the relationship in the room. With any psychological theory, evidence, or knowledge, however, counselling psychologists tend to be concerned with *usefulness* rather than *truth*. Knowledge is only useful when it is useful for understanding *this individual client*, and for helping that client understand themselves.

A counselling psychologist must meet the competencies outlined in the HCPC *Standards of Proficiency* (SOPs) (HCPC, 2015) in order to practice. The HCPC has three levels of standard: standards that all regulated health professionals must meet; generic standards that all practitioner psychologists must meet; and more specific standards that are particular to each type of practitioner psychologist. In order to understand more about counselling psychology in the UK, go to the *Standards of Proficiency* for practitioner psychologists and look at the ones that are specified as "counselling psychologist only". In these, you will be able to discern the things that are most important to the profession: empathy; the importance of language; the role of philosophy; the centrality of the relationship; the need to always consider the client in their context(s); the use of the therapist's self; and the insistence on flexible practice that suits the individual client.

What kinds of people do counselling psychologists work with?

Counselling psychologists work with all types of people. The *Standards of Proficiency* (HCPC, 2015) state that counselling psychologists must "understand psychological models related to a range of presentations including . . . service users with presentations from acute to enduring and mild to severe" (p. 14). One cannot define a counselling psychologist by the population(s) he or she works with, and practitioners may work with everyone from people who are having short-term adjustment issues to an acute crisis, through to severely distressed individuals with long-standing psychological and emotional issues.

While some of the problems that counselling psychologists work with are predominantly psychological/social, including "problems of coping, adaptation and resilience to adverse circumstances and life events, including bereavement and other chronic physical and mental health conditions" (HCPC, 2015, p. 14), counselling psychologists are also expected to understand biological and neuropsychological aspects in clients' presentations. Most counselling psychologists will be equipped through their training and experience to see people from all walks of life, from various social and cultural backgrounds, and of a range of ages; because they are not *required* to undertake training with specific populations, however, counselling psychologists are not professionally obliged to be proficient in working with children, older adults, learning disabilities, and neuropsychological problems. They may always work in these areas if they have the competencies, but it is not usually a core feature of their training.

Course input and placement experiences within counselling psychology tend to emphasise individual work with adults. In an individual's path to qualification, however, he or she may gain experience in many other ways of working. The BPS' standards for doctoral programmes in counselling psychology state that, at the end of their training programmes, counselling psychologists must "be able to provide psychological therapy interventions . . . to individual adults and depending on placement experience other client groups including children and young people, older adults, couples, groups, families and organisations" (BPS, 2015, p. 21). Once again, the scope to design an individually-crafted experience is clear; beyond the baseline competencies required of you, if you have a particular professional area of interest, counselling psychology generally allows you to pursue it.

One of my own doctoral students, for example, had a particular interest in learning disabilities (LD), which is an area that the typical counselling psychology training does not cover in any depth. Luckily, he had professional contacts that enabled him to get an excellent placement in a National Health Service (NHS) LD department. While he had other placement experiences as well over the course of his training, which is essential for counselling psychologists since they are always expected to be able to work with diverse presentations, he fulfilled over half of his required clinical training hours at his LD placement. Given that he also undertook his doctoral research within the area, this trainee developed a specialism in LD that set the course for the rest of his career, and he continues to work successfully in the sector.

Where do counselling psychologists work?

Counselling psychologists work in a wide range of places. In no particular order of popularity or frequency, you can find them employed in hospitals (psychiatric or general, NHS or private); specialist services for particular populations (children and adolescents, older adults, people with learning difficulties); community mental health teams (CMHTs); and a variety of other settings, including forensic settings, corporations, schools, higher education institutions, social services, employee assistance programmes (EAPs), and voluntary organisations of all types. With respect to NHS employment specifically, Table 2.1 shows where counselling psychologists tend to be concentrated across services, based on a survey conducted in June 2016 by the BPS Division of Counselling Psychology. Since many respondents had worked in multiple employments since qualification, the percentages shown in the table do not add up to 100%, but overall this table gives a sense of the breadth of opportunity for counselling psychologists and a sense of the diverse skill sets within the profession.

Counselling psychologists may also be employed as academics, perhaps training the psychologists of the future, as I do, and/or as researchers. A large number of counselling psychologists are also self-employed as

Table 2.1 Counselling psychologists in the NHS

Type of service	Percentage
Adult services	73.4
Community Mental Health Teams (CMHTs)	36.4
Crisis Resolution & Home Treatment (CRHT) services	2.8
Assertive Outreach Teams (AOTs)	0.7
Early Intervention for Psychosis (EIP) services	4.9
Rehabilitation and recovery teams	7.7
Improving Access to Psychological Therapy (IAPT)	25.9
Child & Adolescent Mental Health Services (CAMHS)	16.1
IAPT for children and young people	2.8
Perinatal mental health services	2.1
Forensic services	9.1
Learning Disability (LD) services	7.0
Older adult services	6.3
Memory services	0.7
Substance misuse services	8.4
Physical health psychology services	16.1
Sexual health	4.2
Eating disorder services	10.5

Source: BPS Division of Counselling Psychology membership survey, June 2016, N=143.

independent practitioners, individually or within group practices, working out of their homes or out of separate consulting rooms.

This flexibility with respect to counselling psychologists' work settings begins at – or even before – the training stage. Training courses will accept previous work in a variety of contexts as being relevant to training in counselling psychology. Once formal training placements have commenced, some courses may require that certain types of working environments (e.g., NHS) form part of the overall training, but trainees may choose any clinical placement that fulfills the requirements of the course. Once qualified, counselling psychologists have employment options that extend well beyond the clinical sector – you can choose to work for all or part of your time within academic, organisational, or community contexts, and many counselling psychologists are so-called "portfolio professionals", with many strings to their bow.

Of the counselling psychologists who responded to the June 2016 survey from Table 2.1, 54.2% worked full-time within the NHS, and a further 39.6% worked part-time but spent at least half of their week within NHS services.

Developing the qualities you need to succeed

Any counselling psychologist experiences a great deal of personal and professional growth over their training and their subsequent career. Inevitably, people learn, change, and grow into the profession. An established, experienced counselling psychologist will certainly embody the values of the profession more than a first-year trainee. That said, before you position yourself at the starting line, it is important to think about whether those values resonate with your personality. That resonance is difficult to force or fake, so be honest with yourself: When you read this book, and this chapter, does what I am discussing feel like "home" to you? If it feels like a natural fit, or if at least you aren't dismissing these ideas out of hand, read on to think about the qualities you will need to develop to succeed in training and beyond.

To qualify as a counselling psychologist in the first place, you must have well-developed academic abilities, for the threshold for qualification as a counselling psychologist in the United Kingdom is set at doctoral level or equivalent. This means that you will need to possess or develop strong language skills – in both reading and writing – and the capacity for critical thought and engagement with ideas at a high level. (For more on the doctoral qualities you will need to succeed during training, see the next two chapters.) The doctoral-level abilities to think, notice, and understand are not just critical for success in training, however, as the following paragraph will explain.

The best counselling psychologists have developed sharp, curious, critical, open minds. They are able to track things, to remember things, and to synthesise multiple strands of information. While they possess much knowledge derived from theory and research, they delicately balance this with knowledge derived from the current context, and the individual client embedded in it. They seek to draw out the client's experience, to privilege what is meaningful to the client, and to understand and work from the client's perspective. Their "usefulness rather than truth" perspective is connected to their belief in the existence and salience of multiple truths. In other words, counselling psychologists tend to think and act *pluralistically*, meaning that they are open to many different ways of knowing, and many different kinds of evidence. They hold their own assumptions and knowledge lightly; they are willing to question and challenge established systems or narratives, whether their own or other people's; and they are willing to change their approach in line with evolving understanding.

Experienced and accomplished counselling psychologists have a high level of self-awareness, and a keen sensitivity to the dynamics of relationships. Viewing the relationship as a key vehicle for therapeutic change, counselling psychologists develop an advanced ability to notice and respond to all elements of relating. They attend simultaneously to their own process, the interpersonal process, and the other person's process. They are skilled at *noticing*, and they are likely to be noticing *process* rather than *content* a large portion of the time. They are dedicated to reflexive practice, to noticing and responding to their own perspective; they will be aware of how their "own stuff" might be affecting their work, and they will manage it in a way that facilitates rather than impinges upon the work. Transparency, honesty, humility, and genuineness are key characteristics of a skilled counselling psychologist. In their relationships with clients, they tend to position themselves as committed collaborators rather than as experts or teachers. Personalities who prefer to be in control or in charge, or whose security relies on being an "expert", may find that the counselling psychology ethos is an uneasy fit for them.

What does a career in counselling psychology look like?

As with any profession, counselling psychologists' career paths widen and develop more branches as they move through their careers. Chapter 6 provides a handful of case studies that give a taster of all the possibilities open to you, so please do skip forward if you are curious! Suffice to say, for now, that during the five or so years after qualification as a psychologist, you are still exploring and defining your professional role. As a newly-qualified practitioner, you will likely work in well-supported employment contexts, perhaps within the NHS, voluntary organisations, or private providers of psychological services. NHS jobs have established national pay scales, and a newly-qualified counselling psychologist usually starts within Band 7 on that scale, somewhere between £31,383 and £41,373 depending on experience. If you work in the private sector or independent practice, your income would of course vary depending on your employer and your situation, but in the early phase of your career you might expect it to be roughly similar to the range above. For the latest information on salary prospects for psychologists, check current pay scales on the NHS Employers website or simply search online for "Agenda for Change pay scales".

Of course, if you are in independent/private practice and charging an hourly fee for psychological therapy, you can have quite a lot of control over your hours and rates, and if you wish you can charge whatever the market will bear. Many newly-qualified psychologists wonder whether they should start independent/private practice straightaway, and this is technically possible, although some discourage it because of the extent of support that you may continue to need as a novice professional.

Providing psychological therapy is not the only career option for counselling psychologists, of course – some of us work in academia, training, and/or research. Given their own recent history as trainees, however, many newly-qualified psychologists feel unready to lecture or supervise others, particularly at the doctoral level. On the other hand, some may feel confident to do so; several of my own trainees have taken on part-time posts teaching undergraduate or A-level psychology while they are waiting to become qualified, and some may parlay this into an academic career.

Remember, of course, that it is difficult to speak in terms of a "typical" counselling psychology career, as counselling psychologists often do not limit themselves to any one working context, undertaking multiple part-time jobs rather than one full-time role. These "portfolio careers" can have significant advantages. For example, an employer can provide supportive collegial relationships, annual and parental leave, sick pay, a pension, and other benefits, while a bit of independent practice can provide the flexibility, balance, and autonomy a practitioner might also desire.

As you enter the more "experienced professional" phase, you can expect to start making more deliberate choices, becoming less opportunistic and creating a work role driven by personal values, preferences and priorities. Increased confidence and ability makes successful, enjoyable independent practice more achievable, and many counselling psychologists will incorporate some element of independent practice into their working week even when they are employed elsewhere. As they become more senior, practitioners may move into guiding others in various capacities, becoming managers, senior academics, research supervisors or clinical supervisors. Entrepreneurial activities such as developing one's own service, commissioning, and consulting to organisations, all become possible as expertise deepens. Consultant psychologists in the NHS can find themselves earning on Band 8c or 8d, which means up to £82,434 at time of writing. Up at the top of the pecking order, heads of services can earn up to £99,437.

Various and exciting though these destinations may be, you have to get onto the path if you are ever to reach them. The next chapter will help you think about what you need in order to become the kind of applicant that counselling psychology training courses are seeking. For more experienced practitioners who are considering the independent route, the next chapter will also cover the basic types of background experiences needed to enroll on the BPS' QCoP.

The next step

Equipping yourself for professional training

The savvy traveller knows that the success and smoothness of a journey can depend, to a large extent, on the thoroughness and thoughtfulness of your preparation. A trainee who has prepared well and who is standing on a solid foundation of background experience can endure the slings and arrows of a challenging counselling psychology training far better than their less well-equipped colleagues. But what does good preparation look like? Do you already have what it takes to train? If not, what do you need? Will your undergraduate degree be considered appropriate? Do you have enough work experiences, of the right sort? Is it necessary to undertake any particular courses to make you eligible to apply to study for qualification?

As you will discover, programmes always feature a list of admissions criteria on their websites, including the qualifications and experiences you are meant to have. You may feel like you meet those criteria right now, but take your time to read this chapter. Asked for the best advice they could offer, one programme director said to me, "Tell your readers not to be in a rush to start the training." This is sound counsel, for reasons that I hope will become clear. The next chapter will cover the application process itself, but this chapter is for what comes before – perhaps a significant stretch of time before.

In some places, this chapter might feel as though it gets slightly ahead of itself, for it references both the "taught route" and the "independent route", which are not discussed fully until Chapter 4. Mention of these routes now is essential, however, for how you prepare will depend to some extent on the route you wish to take. For now, however, it is enough to know that taught routes take place on a course with a cohort of peers, whereas the independent route involves training much more autonomously, in a sort of combination of apprenticeship and distance-learning models, under the watchful eye of your Coordinating Supervisor and Placement Supervisors. Whichever your route, however, there is one consideration that overarches and underpins it all, and it is related to the focus of the last chapter:

Make sure you really understand what counselling psychology *is*, and what undertaking a professional training really *means*.

"I know, I know", you may be thinking. "Of course I know!" Are you sure, though? Investigating this thoroughly dramatically reduces your chances of completing a lengthy application on which the personal statement reveals that you are unclear about the profession. You do not want to get to the interview stage before you start to work it out, and this book is designed to give you everything you need to know to ensure that this does not happen to you.

However much you read, there is often no substitute for hearing directly from people who have been there. Throughout this book, some of the most important voices you will hear are from people in the know: programme directors, course leaders, current trainees, and qualified counselling psychologists. The pointers below come straight from the mouths of people in one or more of those positions, who were asked for the best pieces of advice they could give prospective trainees about really understanding the field to which they aspire.

First-year trainee counselling psychologist: *[When preparing to train], because there are so many overlaps, be very clear that you know what clinical psychology is, what counselling psychology is, what counselling is, what psychotherapy is, what a PhD is, what a DPsych is! Be crystal clear about the* combination *of a DPsych and counselling psychology.*

Programme Director, counselling psychology programme: *When an applicant doesn't know what counselling psychology is, when it feels like they just woke up that morning and decided to apply for a doctorate in counselling psychology, it's a big red flag for us. This is a massive personal and professional decision. It's your life. If someone applies to us without understanding the nature of the* *field and the nature of the degree, it makes us wonder whether they are sufficiently mature, responsible and reflexive to undertake the training. It's not about studying up to perform well at the interview. It's about doing thorough research to try and work out if this is what you want to do with your life. If you apply first and do your research about counselling psychology afterwards, I'd go so far as to say that you probably aren't ready.*

First-year trainee counselling psychologist: *I think it was difficult figuring out what counselling psychology was, because, in terms of the work, counselling and clinical psychologists can work in the same settings and do the same type of role. Later on down the road, I realised that a main difference was about a philosophy and a theoretical standpoint, as opposed to the work that you do. I got that on the admissions interviews! You might want to check that out before you go into that process.*

Second-year trainee counselling psychologist: *Do your scoping. Try to draw on as many resources as you can. Gather information from wherever you can: open days, speak to trainees, speak to counselling psychologists.*

I have seen many trainees eagerly begin a course, having aspired to counselling psychology training for ages, only to realise sometime during the first year that they had fundamentally misunderstood what the profession really involves. Getting onto a training programme is a great goal to have, but only if you really understand the object in your sights. I hope that this chapter will help you construct the solid foundation for training that I spoke about; additionally, along the way, it should give you more clarity about whether this type of work is what you really want. The rest of this chapter is divided into four further sections, mapped onto the four key elements of counselling psychology training: academic work, clinical practice, research, and personal development.

Academic experiences

Baseline academic prerequisites for professional training

The bottom line for admission to postgraduate psychology training in the UK is Graduate Basis for Chartership (GBC). This was discussed in Chapter 1 but bears emphasis here. The threshold for this is "an undergraduate honours degree at a minimum lower second class honours level which is accredited by the Society or alternatively an accredited conversion course" (www.bps.org.uk). Although a 2:2 will confer GBC, many training programmes set the bar for admission at 2:1, and you may need to up the ante by doing further study – more on this in the sections below. First, however, let me expend a few more words on GBC, particularly for those who may not be pursuing the most straightforward route to its acquisition.

Without GBC, you will not be able to complete any training that is approved by the BPS, and the rationale for this is perhaps understandable. Any curriculum on a postgraduate psychology training course will be based around the assumption that you already have a foundational Bachelor's degree (Level 6) knowledge of psychology. The postgraduate phase of your education is meant to *develop* your existing psychological knowledge and to train you in its *specialised application*; it will not start from scratch.

When you have GBC, it is safer to assume that you have the requisite depth and breadth of knowledge of psychological theory and practice, and necessary grasp of various research methods, to successfully train at the postgraduate level. If you completed your psychology degree in the more distant past, however, your knowledge may be a bit on the rusty side. To avoid feeling completely lost, you should brush up, at least, and do further formal study, at most. The Quality Assurance Agency for Higher Education publishes a *Subject Benchmark Statement* for psychology that outlines what undergraduate psychology courses in the UK need to cover (QAA, 2010), and this is the standard against which any application for GBC is measured. If it has been a while since you undertook your undergraduate degree, look at the *Subject Benchmark for Psychology*. It might help you target particular areas of knowledge that need refreshing.

Before you start thinking that all undergraduate psychology programmes in the UK conform to the *Subject Benchmark Statement* in precisely the same way, however, let me correct you on that. If you are happening to read this book at an early stage, while you still have a choice of where to undertake your undergraduate study, consider your alternatives carefully. Not all undergraduate psychology programmes are the same, and some will be better set up for later professional training in counselling psychology training than others. An undergraduate course that heavily emphasises traditional, positivist, experimental psychology will feel less relevant, while a programme that actually incorporates counselling training will set you up exceptionally well. In the example below, one qualified counselling psychologist describes the latter sort of undergraduate degree.

> **Early-career qualified counselling psychologist:** *One of the biggest helping factors for me in preparing for counselling psychology training was my undergraduate course. I studied psychology with counselling, where the counselling aspect of the course counted for approximately a quarter of my credits for each of the three years. It was modelled on a counselling diploma. We did "fish bowl" exercises and self-awareness strategies, and every week we had to watch our own recorded therapy practice and hand in process notes. It was fantastic, but many courses today offer only a "light" version of this, I think because it's not as financially valid to take a group of 20 people and do practical skills, compared to taking 80 people and just delivering traditional lectures. Doing that kind of course enabled me to start voluntary counselling whilst still studying, and prepped me well for my doctorate. So for me, choosing your undergraduate course wisely is so necessary and can be the first step to becoming a reflective practitioner.*

Although it seems like a basic thing to remind you about, do ensure that you *can* get GBC before setting your sights on postgraduate training. The most common (and straightforward) way of obtaining GBC is to complete an approved undergraduate psychology degree in the UK (or a UK degree delivered internationally) that meets the benchmarks set out by the QAA. The course described above contained a significant element of counselling, but retained enough psychology to give its graduates GBC. If you are currently enrolled on an undergraduate psychology course, or you are interested in a particular one, go to the British Psychological Society website (www.bps.org.uk) and do an accredited course search. If you have an undergraduate degree in some other field, you can search for a "conversion course" in the same place, or you can look for an appropriate Master's-level training in psychology to give you other core bits of knowledge that will render you eligible for

GBC under the "special-case route". The special-case route provision exists precisely because so many special situations can arise!

As an example of a special situation, people who have studied abroad and/or who are immigrants to the UK may often follow an idiosyncratic, sometimes circuitous route to GBC. GBC applicants from international universities who have done an undergraduate degree in psychology will have their degrees assessed to see whether the content of the degree was roughly similar to UK programmes in breadth and depth; if it is equivalent to at least a 2:2 UK degree (lower second class honours); and if it consisted of at least 50% psychology content. Even if the degree does not quite come up to scratch, one may still be able to apply under the special-case process. If you are someone who has gained one or more psychology degrees outside of the UK, perhaps my own story will help illustrate how the special-case route can work for you – and how important it is to never assume, always assess!

In 1999, I enrolled on a postgraduate training course that was an approved course route towards becoming a BPS-chartered counselling psychologist. I had a BA Hons, so I thought that Graduate Basis for Registration (GBR, as GBC was then known) would be no problem – particularly since I had also completed nearly all the taught components of a four-year professional doctorate in clinical psychology, including 700 client hours' worth of clinical experience. If I had done more research, I might have realised earlier that there could be a problem: all of this education had taken place in the United States, and I had taken a typical American "double major". Because the programme had accepted me without proof of GBR, I didn't think about it until halfway through my course. I then made the discovery about needing 50% undergraduate psychology content. I was two percentage points short, and the BPS was unmoved by my pleas.

On the programme on which I now work, we insist on proof of GBC; alternatively, if someone is completing an undergraduate degree, we make a conditional offer until it is received. Back then, however, I got quite far down the road before realising that I could not reach my intended destination. Gutted, I switched to an MA in Psychotherapy and Counselling so that I didn't lose everything I had done. I had learned the "never assume, always assess" rule the hard way. Eventually, I gained more experience and applied successfully under the special-case process for my chartership and registration as a counselling psychologist, but it was a long and difficult road.

Master's degrees

The vast majority of counselling psychology training programmes do not require you to have a Master's degree as a condition for entry. Instead, the first year of the doctorate is considered to be Master's level (Level 7), moving on to doctoral level (Level 8) in Year 2 and beyond. So the fact that you need not get a Master's before embarking on professional training in counselling psychology is good news – or is it? Once again, the experiences of actual counselling psychology trainees, shown below, give us a few things to think about.

> **Second-year trainee counselling psychologist:** *From undergraduate, I really noticed the jump. If you're passionate about it, it's doable, but you have to be so interested and so determined! I was stretched particularly in terms of criticality, and in terms of originality of thought. The ability to write "I think" or "in my opinion" was something that was not even toyed with at undergrad!*

> **Second-year trainee counselling psychologist:** *It was reassuring for me knowing that there was an M-level inset into the first year. I thought, "okay, there's an exit award after a year or so, and then there's a D-level". I think I experienced a jump the first year from undergraduate to the first year of the M-level, rather than M-level to D-level.*

> **Second-year trainee counselling psychologist:** *I don't know whether this applies always, but I feel like it was D-level that we were marked at in the first year! (laughs) We were taught by counselling psychologists who were just used to teaching at doctoral level, so I haven't noticed the jump between first and second year. That made me curious as to how much of an M-level we were really being marked at in the first year!*

> **Nearly-qualified trainee counselling psychologist:** *I spent at least the first year and a half of the course feeling out of my depth. I was almost the only person without a Master's, and really worried that I wouldn't make the grade academically. Actually, I did make the*

grade – but more experience before I started would have made the first year less harrowing for me.

Second-year trainee counselling psychologist: *I had done a Master's before, and I was amazed at the jump between that Master's and starting this course. I think it was the highest academic jump I've noticed. How to help manage that? Do your reading, be interested in what it is you're doing, and ask for help when you need it.*

As you can see, trainees often feel shocked at, and unprepared for, the level of academic study on a doctoral programme. To better prepare yourself, therefore, and to compete with others applying for professional training, you might wish to consider the benefits of a Master's degree even in those instances where it is not required. The successful completion of a relevant Master's degree may also be the only way that a training programme will consider you if you have less than a 2:1 for your undergraduate. Beginning in 2016, the government began offering postgraduate loans for UK residents at UK universities, making Master's degrees more accessible.

Undertaking a Master's-level degree in any subject will better prepare you for tackling the next level up, but it will of course be helpful to you if the Master's is in a relevant discipline. If your ultimate aim is to become a counselling psychologist, what is the best choice? You could situate yourself within psychology more broadly by doing a psychology MSc or PGDip "conversion course"; focus on an allied branch of psychology, so as to form the basis of an eventual additional professional qualification; or do an M-level degree in psychotherapy or counselling.

Conversion courses in psychology primarily cater to those who do not have an accredited undergraduate degree in psychology, and who need an additional degree to acquire GBC; however, many of them purport to go beyond the "core" material required and position themselves as offering a stepping-stone between undergraduate and doctoral training. Accredited conversion courses tend to be Postgraduate Diplomas or MSc degrees, the latter of which is likely to involve a more significant element of research. "Psychology", "Psychological Sciences", or "Psychological Studies" may be in the title of the degree. For someone whose undergraduate education was in the more distant past, or who wants exposure to more research or to M-level studies generally before moving on to a professional doctorate, a conversion course may be quite suitable even if you already have GBC.

If, in addition to your interest in counselling psychology, you are drawn to another practitioner psychology, you may wish to consider an M-level degree in that discipline. In addition to conferring knowledge and orientation to M-level study, it could also assist you down the line. In many branches of applied psychology, becoming registered involves an M-level training programme on a course route *plus* two years of supervised practice via a "Stage 2" BPS qualification. (Contact the Qualifications office at the BPS for more information or see the Careers portal on www.bps.org.uk for more information.) Acquiring multiple practitioner psychologist registrations is always possible for those who meet the training requirements and standards, and if you would like to maximise your opportunities, undertaking a Master's in an allied psychological discipline would set you up well.

"Why not just undertake an MSc or MA in Counselling Psychology?", you might be wondering. When psychology became regulated by the HCPC, the threshold for qualification for some practitioner psychologists was set at doctoral- rather than Master's-level – in other words, educational, clinical, and counselling psychologists must now undertake a doctoral-level qualification to qualify for the register and to use the protected titles associated with these professions. As a consequence, there are fewer standalone degrees out there that actually term themselves "MSc/MA in Counselling Psychology", and most have changed their titles to avoid veering into protected-title territory. If you see a degree entitled "Master's in Psychological Counselling" or "Master's in Therapeutic Counselling", however, this might be an excellent preparation for your eventual doctoral training.

Finally, many counselling psychology training courses require you to have undertaken formal counselling skills training (more on this in the next section on "clinical experience"). While the admissions panel on a taught course will not require your previous counselling training to be a more academic MA or MSc, if you want to combine the experience of Master's-level work with a deeper understanding of counselling theory and practice, and avail yourself of the opportunity to try your hand at higher-level research and academic writing, this could be just the ticket.

Both the British Association for Counselling and Psychotherapy (BACP, www.bacp.co.uk) and the United Kingdom Council for Psychotherapy (UKCP, www.psychotherapy.org.uk) keep lists of accredited MA and

MSc programmes. See their websites for details of those courses, as well as their official publications (such as the BACP's monthly magazine, *Therapy Today*). Master's programmes may go by many different names, whether generic (e.g., MA in Counselling, MA in Psychotherapy & Counselling) or specific (e.g., MA in Person-Centred Experiential Counselling & Psychotherapy).

People who take the independent route to qualification as a counselling psychologist have to submit evidence that they have met a number of requirements, to include competencies in psychotherapy and in research. Here is where having experienced formal study on a Master's will significantly help you on your way! The current Registrar for the QCoP explains more below, and highlights why the type of Master's you do, and the type of research you have done on it, can be important.

Dr Victoria Galbraith, C.Psychol., Registered Counselling Psychologist and Registrar for the QCoP: *The advice I always give is that, if you are taking a course to prepare you for training as a counselling psychologist, consider doing it to Master's level, and consider a Master's in counselling and psychotherapy, which may tick the "core therapy training" box, but which may also tick the research dissertation box, as long as it has counselling, psychotherapy, or counselling psychology underpinnings to the research project. Some people may come into the QCoP with a Master's degree in something, psychology for instance, and they will have done a research project as part of that. If that project didn't have the* therapeutic *side to it, when that unit is eventually assessed on the QCoP, the candidate will have to write a persuasive 5,000-word piece explaining how it applies to counselling psychology.*

A Master's can help you meet requirements for the research-related requirements of the QCoP, and this can be a real bonus for individuals pursuing the independent route. Because they must be so much more autonomous than their course-route peers, arranging a significant research project can be quite a bit harder from their position of relative independence. Any candidate on the QCoP who has undertaken a formal M-level degree in the past will be in a much better position to hit the ground running.

Counselling and psychotherapy training

As noted earlier, many (although not all) training programmes in counselling psychology require applicants to have undertaken formal training in counselling skills. Such courses tend to have a vocational focus, which means they will feel quite different from a more academically orientated Master's. The moment you start looking into the possibilities, you might notice yourself feeling slightly overwhelmed. The content, structures, frequencies and durations of counselling trainings vary tremendously, and you will find plenty of opportunities to just dip your toe in the water, committing just a few days or weeks.

To best prepare you for counselling psychology training, however, it may be wisest to undertake something a bit more substantial, at a higher level of the UK's Regulated Qualifications Framework (RQF). Visit the National Careers Service section of www.direct.gov.uk to review the qualifications table there. Counselling trainings at lower levels will still be useful, and if you have limited time you may wish to access whatever you can, but the most solid preparation for training will come from Level 7 programmes of study in counselling or psychotherapy, which will naturally follow on from, and build upon, your Bachelor's-level degree The trainees below talk about why counselling skills training helped them.

First-year trainee counselling psychologist: *For me the foundation course orientated me to the different models and gave me the practice of counselling, but it was also about having experience on a course. It was also an opportunity to sort some of my own stuff out before I got on the course! . . . and because that is such a core part of being a counselling psychologist, I think if you can get a head start, that's the real benefit of doing a foundation course as well.*

First-year trainee counselling psychologist: *I did the Level 3 Certificate in Counselling Studies, and I also did a certificate in counselling in Sri Lanka, which was really interesting! The first one was very regulated and the Sri Lanka one was not regulated at all, but to have that diversity and that knowledge and to see how therapists approach the client differently was literally mind-blowing.*

Third-year trainee counselling psychologist: *Academically, I don't think I learnt much from my counselling certificate – probably* *not a good thing to say! Ours didn't have much in the way of skills either. But importantly, it helped me begin to critique my interactions, particularly professionally, and to reflect.*

Nearly-qualified trainee counselling psychologist: *The foundation course made me really curious and also excited about working clinically. But it was also quite scary because it suddenly sinks in that you are working with real people and real problems, and that you want to be really careful. It puts a lot of responsibility on you. It dawned on me what a huge undertaking counselling psychology training is.*

As can be seen from the testimonials above, undertaking a foundation course in counselling is not just about acquiring skills. For these trainees, their foundation courses prepared them for counselling psychology training in a different way as well – a deeper, more meaningful level. Additionally, it goes without saying that foundational training in counselling and psychotherapy can be particularly important when you have less of the kind of formal counselling experience that is discussed in the next section.

Clinical experiences

Of all the things that preoccupy and worry applicants to counselling psychology programmes, the extent and nature of their existing experience is probably the most significant. Admissions criteria that seem precise at first blush – such as the common requirement "At least one year of formal one-to-one helping experience" – become muddier the more one thinks about them. The question of whether five hours of helpline work a week for the last three years constitutes "at least one year" may keep you at your calculator for a while. And what does "formal" mean? Does telephone experience count? What if you've only done groupwork? Does befriending, mentoring, or teaching count as the right kind of "formal helping experience"? What if you have shadowed a psychologist or otherwise worked in the right kinds of settings, but you have not personally provided services to clients? What if you have worked as a research assistant in a psychology department, which must surely count as relevant somehow, but not as a counsellor?

The bottom line is, programmes need you to have experience of a psychological or psychotherapeutic nature, and the more "formal" that experience is – that is, the more it looks like substantial experience of one-to-one counselling sessions with individual, real-world clients – the better off you are. Not all one-to-one work is created equal, however. Befriending and mentoring activities, for example, do involve one-to-one relationships, intended to support and encourage people who are isolated, at risk, or otherwise vulnerable. These tend to be viewed as less relevant, however, perhaps because the nature and boundaries of such interactions differ so significantly from therapeutic relationships, and some programmes even emphasise that your experience should go "beyond befriending". Furthermore, you may have spent considerable time in psychological, psychotherapeutic, or medical environments, but it matters quite a lot what you did there. You may have shadowed qualified professionals, or otherwise assisted their work in some capacity. You may have worked in clerical, administrative, or other roles. In both of these situations you may have gained a lot of knowledge through osmosis and observation, but programmes are likely to view this as too indirect to be considered sufficiently relevant experience.

Below is a selection of clinical experiences that some of my own trainees had at the point of applying for training on a course that required "one year (or equivalent) clinical experience".

- One year of hospice telephone line, providing breast cancer support; facilitator of meditation and stress-relief workshops.

- Four years of volunteer work and 10 years of full-time employment in drug services with multiple comorbid problems.

- Support work with autistic children; inclusion support worker for young people; five years of IAPT work as PWP and group facilitator.

- One to two days a week as voluntary assistant psychologist in the NHS for one year; six-month research assistantship; volunteer work on a mental-health helpline.

- Psychology teacher for two years; independent counselling; counsellor on an Employee Assistance Programme.

- Part-time befriender at Mind; support work with National Autistic Society; mentor with university students; research work; voluntary part-time assistant psychologist post for one year.

- Groupwork in a social-working setting with addiction; counselling with expats while overseas; wellbeing manager; existential-phenomenological psychotherapist.
- Voluntary work in inpatient drug and alcohol setting and eating disorders service.
- Seven months volunteering in dementia day-care centre and seven months volunteer work with mental health charity.

But what if you have little clinical experience to speak of, and still want to apply for training? Certainly, many different "nonclinical" work and life experiences may contribute to your readiness for training, and much depends on how you position yourself during the application process. The stories below show that for some individuals who were able to make their case well, the worst-case scenario – not having any formal one-to-one counselling experience – did not ultimately prove a barrier to accessing professional training, even if it caused some difficulty further down the line.

Third-year trainee counselling psychologist: *My most significant preparation came in the form of midwifery training and then working as a midwife. Although not directly related to psychology, the clinical experience of working with a huge variety of families and being integrated into the NHS was invaluable and will help direct the path I hope to take towards working with women and families as a psychologist when I qualify. I also gained valuable experience with documentation and record-keeping, working within a code of practice and understanding some of the universal challenges faced by NHS staff.*

Early-career qualified counselling psychologist: *I did not have any counselling experience. I had, however, become a coordinator of a parents' network to do with my daughter's disability. I found that I enjoyed helping other parents, listening to them and giving them hope. I then took up a voluntary position as a Home Start volunteer in preparation. This was quite strategic, as I figured that I needed to have had some kind of experience when applying.*

First-year trainee counselling psychologist: *I had little formal experience of one-to-one counselling as such. I'd done a lot of mentoring and one-to-one teaching, and in my application and interview* *attempted to demonstrate that these applications (and the length of time doing them) were a good enough base layer to build skills on to from classes. Who you are is as important as the experience you have. So, I would say, don't let a lack of formal experience put you off applying; think carefully about your character and attributes with people and how this can be demonstrated.*

Qualified counselling psychologist: *I had worked with vulnerable people but had no one-to-one counselling experience when I started on the course. The first two years of training felt like a roller-coaster ride. It was very hard on me.*

First-year trainee counselling psychologist: *I had done coaching and executive coaching, tutoring, mentoring for tutors and students, befriending with vulnerable older adults, and another befriending with LD patients in a care home. I've done 15 years' worth of stuff, but it wasn't the right stuff. Before I started the course, I should have done six months as a volunteer counsellor. That would have made it so much easier, because finding a placement has been so much angst.*

What is clear from the stories above is that training courses *do* accept people with a variety of professional experiences, even when the admissions criteria emphasise formal counselling experience. Once on the course, however, less experienced people may encounter a greater level of difficulty in the competitive clinical placements market, and the last story highlights the drawbacks, relatively speaking, of possessing mostly befriending and mentoring type experience. Once on a course and seeking placements, more experienced individuals will have the edge not only because of their CV, but because of the existing networking connections they have. This is not the only consideration, however. A professional training in counselling psychology involves learning curves in multiple arenas – academic, clinical, research, and personal development. When the clinical learning curve is less steep, the degree of exhaustion becomes correspondingly less!

So, how can you obtain the kind of clinical experience that will not only help you access training, but will be most helpful once you are on a course? First of all, even though many organisations will provide training before you are let loose on real service users, consider first getting the kind of counselling training described in an earlier section – this will make you more confident, more skilled, and more "employable". Even voluntary counselling and helpline posts are limited in number and choosy in their selection processes. If you decide to undertake course-based training, you will likely see opportunities advertised in your place of study. Although some of these might be restricted to people on particular degree programmes, do make inquiries.

All that having been said, let us think about two work contexts for gaining helping experience – the voluntary sector, and the NHS.

Voluntary sector experiences

Volunteer counselling and active-listening opportunities are relatively easy to find, if you are looking in the right places, and especially if you have already undertaken counselling training. Search for work on www. bacp.co.uk, in the back pages of magazines like *Therapy Today*, and through Internet search engines (try plugging in "volunteer counselling placements"). While there may be some opportunities with smaller charities, you may wish to investigate large, nationwide organisations with recognisable names and multiple locations, which tend to have established training programmes for volunteer counsellors and helpline volunteers.

The types of opportunities at the organisations listed below vary considerably, and some do require a certain level of qualification or experience for the more "formal" counselling roles. While some offer face-to-face experience, others involve helpline work. Some construe volunteers' work as "active listening" rather than counselling (especially on helplines), but even active listening work can be good experience. Read the volunteer job descriptions carefully to get a better sense, and have a look at the training offered, as this too will be valuable for your CV. These examples are not provided as particular recommendations for places to pursue, but represent a selection of organisations that appear frequently on counselling psychology applicants' CVs.

- Mind (www.mind.org.uk)
- Samaritans (www.samaritans.org)
- NSPCC/ChildLine (www.nspcc.org.uk)
- Cruse Bereavement Care (www.cruse.org.uk)

- Place2Be (www.place2be.org.uk)
- Anxiety UK (www.anxietyuk.org.uk)
- Age UK (www.ageuk.org.uk).

Working in the National Health Service

Competition for assistant psychologist posts in the NHS is notoriously intense, even though the type and quality of the experience you will get varies tremendously by post. On one end of the spectrum, you could serve as a glorified administrative assistant, but on the other, you could find yourself managing a large caseload of people with complex difficulties. You may garner substantial experience of research, clinical audits, and/or service evaluation, or you may be exposed to none of these. When perusing jobs on *The Psychologist* website (probably the best place to look for such posts), make sure you read the job description thoroughly to get a sense of what you would be doing, and assess carefully whether it fits with what you want and need.

Another option in the NHS is working as a Psychological Wellbeing Practitioner (PWP), which many of my own trainees did before entering the programme. The PWP role forms part of the Improving Access to Psychological Therapies (IAPT) programme, which is currently a major feature of the mental health landscape in the UK. As such, exposure to the IAPT system as a PWP is not only a good way of gaining experience prior to training, but can also be a savvy investment in your future career. PWPs perform many so-called "low-intensity" activities that are excellent preparation for professional training as a practitioner psychologist: they assist people with guided self-help; help them manage their medications; case-manage referrals; signpost to other organisations; assess for psychological problems; and work on treatment plans that are both personalised and evidence-based. Work as a PWP requires approximately one year training part-time, and a list of accredited training courses can be accessed on www.bps.org.uk/pwp.

Most counselling psychology trainers would advise you to undertake relevant, good-quality work experience *before* deciding that this is what you want to do, not just as a way of getting onto a training programme. If you are just finishing an undergraduate qualification, think carefully about whether you are really ready to apply. Give yourself time to gain meaningful, substantive experience – you will be far better prepared.

Research experiences

In the backgrounds of some of the trainees below, you may notice research experience. Even though qualifying as a counselling psychologist in the UK involves a professional doctorate rather than a PhD, research and inquiry will form a major component of your training. Trainees on both the independent and taught routes will need to demonstrate all of the research competencies outlined by the BPS (see Section 6 of the *Standards for the Accreditation of Doctoral Programmes in Counselling Psychology*, BPS, 2015). Additionally, particularly on a taught route, trainees must produce a piece of research that meets the doctoral hallmarks of originality and contribution to the field (QAA, 2008). It is a high bar to hit, and the more research experience you have ahead of doctoral training, the easier it will be to reach.

Counselling psychology is a methodologically pluralistic field, and qualified professionals are expected to be familiar with a range of approaches to research and inquiry. In order to use and understand existing research in the field, and to be able to carry out original research, counselling psychologists need to have a sound working knowledge of all sorts of research methods, and trainees' research projects may be quantitative, qualitative, or pragmatically multi-strategy, depending on the research question. In my experience, most trainees who have really struggled – and who have fallen down – were mostly tripped up by the research element.

Once upon a time, applicants for training underestimated the importance of research and tended to neglect this aspect of their pre-training development, but clearly, this is no longer possible. Interview panels are now far keener to assess research capability, sometimes requesting that applicants submit research proposals. "It's great when [applicants] can demonstrate research-mindedness", says one faculty member on a doctoral programme. "This does not mean they need to have their doctoral research project sorted, but that they can demonstrate interest in research and can talk about any previous research they have done coherently." Another trainer who works with multiple counselling psychology programmes puts it more strongly: "If you've never thought of what kind of research you might want to do for your doctoral thesis, go away and don't come back until you have!" Clearly, the "doctoral culture" has been growing within counselling psychology ever since the HCPC set the threshold at the doctoral level, and the word is spreading. As at least some of the testimonials below show, aspirant counselling psychologists are increasingly aware that research is a key element.

> **First-year trainee counselling psychologist:** *I'm here because of the research. I knew what area I wanted to research when I came. When I was choosing the course, that's also what it was about.*

> **First-year trainee counselling psychologist:** *It's been a challenge to try and come up with a research topic. At first I was thinking about something fast and easy, but as I've learned more, I'm thinking: what really interests me? What do I really want to know more about?*

> **First-year trainee counselling psychologist:** *In all honesty, when I first thought about applying, I thought research was something I would have to do to get the doctorate and practice. On open days I had the message about research hammered home, and it opened my eyes to the benefits. Now I would say I'm equally interested in both. If I still thought of it as something I'd have to do, I don't see how I'd survive the course.*

> **Nearly-qualified trainee counselling psychologist:** *At one point I thought about trying for a research career, but my voluntary work, listening and talking to people in emotional distress, was something that used all of me – my emotions, my imagination, my presence – in a way that research didn't. So by the end of my conversion course, counselling psychology – both research and being with people – seemed like a natural goal.*

Despite the positivity expressed in many of the accounts above, research remains a focal point for trainee anxiety. Many deal with this by doggedly avoiding it. I would encourage any aspiring counselling psychologists to remove their heads from the sand and to embrace the idea that research can be an exciting part of their training and career. Read about research in counselling psychology. Strongly consider attending the Division of Counselling Psychology annual conference, which usually happens in July. This event will expose you to the breadth of counselling psychology research, as well as its priorities and values; it will convey something of the current themes and trends in research and practice; it will afford unparalleled networking opportunities; and it will provide further clarity on whether counselling psychology seems like a suitable career path for you.

Because certain training programmes require you to submit a draft research proposal, we will talk about research again in the next chapter, but what's useful to note now is that the level of coherence and persuasiveness in that research proposal will very much depend on your grasp of the essentials of research. Refresh your existing knowledge and extend your understanding by reading books that cover a variety of research designs (e.g., Robson, 2015) and that cover the whole of the research process (e.g., Vossler & Moller, 2015).

Personal experiences

The arenas of experience we have discussed thus far are relatively concrete: there are books you can read, courses you can attend, voluntary placements you can secure, client hours you can log, and open evenings you can attend. The last category is more elusive. It has to do with your level of maturity, with your openness to experience, and with a collection of other qualities that are associated with the profession. Some individuals possess such qualities naturally, irrespective of age and background; others have acquired those qualities through doing "work on themselves", whether through formal personal therapy or not. In the accounts below, both trainers and trainees attempt to capture something of this category of preparation.

> **First-year trainee counselling psychologist:** *I think what really helped me was going to a few sessions of personal therapy. I found it more useful than any course, any reading that I'd done.*

> **Third-year trainee counselling psychologist:** *For me, certain difficult life experiences (for example, being a young carer, difficult break-ups, struggling with feeling "good enough") were very helpful in terms of the placement aspect of training. I believe that having certain "touchstones", which could be used to empathise with clients, made*

me a better therapist and provided me with a sense of confidence and direction in the therapy room.

Early-career qualified counselling psychologist: *We have a lot of diversity amongst CoPs in terms of cultural/racial background, gender, disability, age, and so forth. Struggling with adjustment to another sociocultural environment, encountering prejudice and stereotypes, dealing with health issues . . . I wonder if these experiences are a more personal "preparation" for becoming a counselling psychologist, being more in touch with vulnerability, with existential struggles.*

First-year trainee counselling psychologist: *In my teens and 20s, I was wrapped up in a world of heavy drug and alcohol use and crime. I was in young offender's institutions, rehab, and finally prison. I was allowed out one day a week to study on a basic counselling skills course. After release, I completed a follow-up certificate in counselling, then went travelling for three years, which was invaluable in terms of the person I've become today. After working professionally for several years, I returned to India for a Vipassana ten-day silent meditation retreat, and made some great progress in terms of what it is I wanted to achieve in my life and what was holding me back. Upon returning to the UK I got myself immediately into therapy with a relational psychodynamic therapist. It was shortly after this that I encountered "counselling psychology" as a field and became excited about this as a possible career.*

First-year trainee counselling psychologist: *For me, it's not about a particular personal "experience" or the type/quality of them. When I read the application process and criteria, I began to notice how the products of my experiences – adversities, challenges, gritted teeth, decisions, perseverance, successes – resonated with what the profession was all about. That was ultimately what convinced me to apply.*

Course leader, counselling psychology programme: *I've seen very young people who are quite mature and reflective and have had some life experiences individuals 20 years older haven't had yet. You cannot be ageist in that respect. An older person is more likely to have had more important life experience, but that doesn't necessarily mean that a younger person wouldn't.*

What seems to be highlighted above is that there is no magic formula, and that even if there were one, it would not be related to being any particular age, having done any particular things, being of any particular background. What does seem to be important is something in the following territory. You have learned, but you know that there is always more to learn, and you want to learn it. You have reflected on yourself and your experience, but you realise how important it is that you never stop reflecting. Many things may have happened to you – some of them quite challenging things – but you have managed to stay open to experience, even quite difficult experience, and you are able to sit with others through theirs. Whatever your age, whatever your background, you are ready, and open, and willing.

Having read and reflected on this chapter, ask yourself: "Am I ready?" If the answer is no, take one step at a time. Make your plans, marshall your resources, and do what needs to be done. If it's yes, read on, and get ready to start your training!

4 Becoming a trainee

So, here we are. Having contemplated, researched and prepared, you are poised to take whatever action is necessary to become a trainee counselling psychologist. This chapter supports you from this moment of readiness and intention through to the end of your training. It will guide you through the application process; help you understand what training programmes are looking for; and orientate you to the some of the realities of life as a trainee, including finding clinical placements.

The first two sections of this chapter – "Applying for training" and "Life as a trainee" – are each split into subsections, covering the taught route and independent routes separately. These two pathways to qualification look and feel rather different, and you are encouraged to read through both subsections, bracketing your preconceptions and considering which path seems to suit you and your circumstances best. Many people, accustomed to traditional university-type education structures, are completely unaware of the Qualification and of the fact that, if they wish and if it works for them, they could begin this path straightaway after obtaining their GBC. Rather confusingly, although the independent route does not result in conferral of a doctoral *degree*, it is considered to be doctoral *level*, and it entitles you to HCPC registration as a counselling psychologist, just as the taught route does. So, keep an open mind! It should also be acknowledged that these two paths are not mutually exclusive, as many an independent route candidate has started as a taught-route trainee but changed in response to shifting circumstances. The final section of the chapter deals with one of the most important parts of your training – clinical placement.

Applying for training

Applying on the taught route to qualification

Which programme?

The concept of a taught route to qualification will probably be the most familiar, easily-graspable one for most people. At the time of writing there are 13 HCPC-approved, BPS-accredited taught routes to qualification as a counselling psychologist in the United Kingdom – you will want to consult the HCPC and BPS websites for the most up-to-date information. Naturally, one of the first factors you will consider is *location*. How you do decide where to apply?

Some courses may be more convenient for you geographically, but consider location as balanced against *structure*. While all of the training programmes listed must meet the same broad criteria to receive the stamp of approval from the BPS and the HCPC, the ways in which they are delivered vary significantly. Some require you to be on campus for one or two days per week, extending over three or four years. Others start out with more intensive attendance (two or even three days per week), shifting later on to spending relatively more time with clinical placements or engaged in independent study and research, and less time attending classes. Still others are quite flexibly structured, enabling trainees to attend on a less frequent and/or a flexible basis. These latter training courses in particular may include intensive weeks or weekends alongside some elements of distance learning, and may incorporate significant engagement with the virtual learning environment (VLE). Part-time training is sometimes available – for instance, some courses allow you to split the M-level phase of the course over two years – but other institutions only offer a full-time option. In the interests of future-proofing this book somewhat and not promoting any one course over another, current details of the various courses' structures are not provided here. You are, however, strongly recommended to be systematic about trying to work out which course is best for you.

Try to set considerations of geography and logistics aside for one moment – you never know, commuting or even moving might be the best option if there is a course that you really want. When I was under-taking my own counselling psychology training in London, one of my colleagues commuted from North Wales! Keeping an open mind, set up a table or spreadsheet and enter the websites of all of the available counselling psychology programmes – check the list of accredited pro-grammes on www.bps.org.uk. Create columns for "course location" and "course structure". How is your life set up at the moment? Are you on your own and free to move about as you please? Do you have family? Dependents? Children, other family members, or pets who need you to be there at particular times? Any professional doctoral training is a big undertaking, and getting it to work alongside other commitments in your life is challenging at the best of times. While all training courses are tough, and while not all of the challenges posed to work and family life will be directly related to the hours of work involved or the ways in which those hours are structured, some programmes may be a better fit for your personal circumstances than others.

Be as honest with yourself as possible when looking at the course structures. You may wish to power through and find a course that would enable you to be done and dusted within three years, but this may incur other costs to you. You may like the idea of a course that ena-bles you to attend intensively at weeks or during the evenings, but how will this affect you and other people in your life, and are you indulging in a (probably doomed) fantasy that you will be able to work full-time while you are training?

This latter question brings us to another factor in your decision-making: *financial commitment*. Add another column to your spreadsheet – approximate annual tuition. (The website for each training programme should show this information fairly clearly, but contact the admissions department if you are unclear.) It will quickly become apparent that as well as being costly in terms of time, pursuing the taught route to qualification will have an impact on your bank balance. Although trainee and qualified CoPs work alongside clinical psychologists in the health service, at the time of writing the NHS funds only clinical psychological training. Annual costs of a full-time course vary, and tuition can be significantly more for students who come from outside the European Union. While counselling psychologist trainees often fund their own training, loans, bursaries, scholarships, and/or financial hardship tuition relief may be available depending on the individual's personal situation and the extent of their initiative. Always check with an individual training programme for any special funding available.

Tuition, of course, is not the only cost associated with training. Add another column into your spreadsheet to estimate additional annual costs. See Table 4.1 for an example training-costs calculation for someone who lives in London and who is considering training there as well.

There will be some additional costs, to include professional liability insurance at the trainee rate, if your placement's insurance does not cover you; membership of the BPS and the Division of Counselling Psychology, again charged at the trainee rate; criminal records checks, if this is not provided by your placement or your programme; and any books or other training materials you need or want to purchase.

As you can see in Table 4.1, the cost of counselling psychology training goes beyond tuition and can vary considerably; factors like different requirements for personal therapy, and the amount of private supervision that you may need to undertake if your clinical placement does not offer enough, can have a massive impact on your overall costs. The aspiring counselling psychology trainee in this example clearly lives close enough to Programme A to bike or walk there, eliminating transport expenses, but the personal therapy costs are relatively punchy, and this trainee will end up paying £12,000 over the course of the programme if they feel sufficiently committed to undertaking therapy with their preferred practitioner, who in this example is charging a central-London type rate without a trainee discount. Programme C's lower personal therapy requirement will reduce costs, but is further away, so ultimately the rail costs combined with the four-year nature of the programme actually make it the most expensive option.

Given the expense of training, it is not surprising that many applicants ask the interview panel whether it is possible to hold down paid employment while they are training. Looking at course schedules, this might seem theoretically possible, especially since there are no courses that require Monday-to-Friday attendance. Given the other commitments involved in training, however – clinical placements, supervision, personal therapy, reading, coursework, and research – full-time really does mean full-time. Some of the most stressed trainees I encounter are those attempting to hold down a significant level of paid employment during their counselling psychology course. Rather than assuming that

Table 4.1 Sample training costs worksheet

Programme	Annual tuition/overall cost of training	Private supervision (75 hours over course of training)	Personal therapy	Travel costs	Estimated total cost of training
Programme A	$(£10,350 \times 3)$ + £2,000 thesis submission = £33,050	£65 × 75 for supervisor A = £4,875 £50 × 75 for supervisor B = £3,750 *Note: Check whether I need this much privately or can I get some in-house at placement(s) ... **budget for £4,000***	40 hours per year required – 120 hours £100 per hour for preferred therapist – £12,000 *(Eeek! – check if there's a trainee rate)* £55 per hour at therapist B's trainee rate – £6,600	None – bike or walk from home	**£49,050** if preferred therapist – **£43,650** if I go with therapist B trainee rate
Programme B	£9,500 × 3 = £28,500	See above – budget £4,000	40 hours required for whole course – £4,000 for preferred therapist £2,200 at therapist B's trainee rate	Zone 1–2 annual travelcard £904/year £2,712 total *Check whether I need a travelcard since not there every day!*	**£39,212** if go with preferred therapist **£37,412** if therapist B
Programme C	£6,880 (Y1) + £8,600 (Y2) + £9,460 (Y3) + £8,600 (Y4) = £33,540	See above – budget £4,000	20 hours per year/60 hours total £6,000 for preferred therapist £3,300 for therapist B	Zone 1–9 annual travelcard £2,356/year £9,424 total *Check whether I need a travelcard – not there every day*	**£52,964** for preferred therapist **£50,264** for therapist B

you will be able to maintain both the course and paid employment, consider the following, on a theoretical basis: If you *had* to give up substantive paid employment for three or four years, is there any way you would you be able to? Would savings, loans, gifts, and/or household income enable you to make ends meet? If you research all of the possibilities and the answer to that question is still "no way", consider whether this is the right time for you, or whether the potentially more flexible QCoP option might suit you better (see next section).

From the perspective of the bottom line, Programme B in Table 4.1 looks like the obvious choice, and yet some additional expense might be worth it if Programme B is the course you really want. Every training programme in counselling psychology requires "in depth critical knowledge and supervised clinical experience of the particular theory and practice of at least one specific model of psychological therapy" and "working knowledge and supervised clinical experience of at least one further model of psychological therapy" (British Psychological Society, 2015, p. 21), but these models differ across programmes. Even though all counselling psychology training encompasses a variety of models, a programme with existential-phenomenological therapy as its core model will have a different feel from a programme anchored in psychodynamic or cognitive-behavioural approaches.

Training courses in counselling psychology are a three- to six-year commitment, depending on the structure you choose, and it is important to orientate yourself as much as possible to the core and working models on the various programmes, in service of finding the best fit. While you can get a sense of this through reading, having conversations with different practitioners, and attending personal therapy, there is probably no substitute for doing that certificate course in counselling before applying for training, and even a short-term course can provide clarity. "I went on a week-long counselling course", says one first-year counselling psychology trainee, "and it was doing each specific type of framework, like CBT one day, psychodynamic another day, and so forth. The one I thought I *would* like, I didn't like, and the one I thought I *wouldn't* like, I actually enjoyed." These surprises had quite a meaningful impact on the courses this trainee applied for, and set him on the path to the one he ultimately undertook. So, add another column to that spreadsheet of programmes: core model(s) and working model(s). A difference of £10,000 for the overall training is significant, this is true, but the price of undertaking extensive core training in a model that does not feel right for you may feel much higher.

The particular core and working models on a programme are not the only factors to consider when searching out the right programme for you, however. Courses will differ on a number of other dimensions, and this has its advantages, as argued in the BPS' *Standards for the Accreditation of Doctoral Programmes in Counselling Psychology* (2015).

> Counselling psychology programmes will vary in the emphases they place on work with particular clinical groups, therapeutic modalities, curriculum content, non-therapy skills, training methods etc. This is healthy and promotes diversity and richness within the profession. It ensures programmes can be responsive to regional and national priorities, opens up opportunities for some programmes to coordinate and complement their efforts and offers prospective applicants choice of programmes which best suit their own preferences, learning style and goals.
>
> (p. 18)

People tend to try and get a feel for programmes from websites, from prospectuses, and from open days, but there are other ways to work out what might be right for you. In the example below, one early-career qualified counselling psychologist pulls various threads together – location, feel, other practical considerations – in describing how she identified which courses would work for her.

> **Early-career qualified counselling psychologist:** *I needed to find a training course that had a part-time option due to my childcare commitments, so this excluded a number of them. I also wanted to go somewhere as close as possible to where I lived. I identified two universities and attended open days at both, which was important. One of them I ruled out following an introductory weekend, as it did not feel as grounded in psychology as the other course; I also did not like the place it was housed in, which was not very university-like. To me, the academic side was as important as the psychotherapeutic side.*
>
> *Every counselling psychology training course has a different culture, a different style, a different emphasis. You can only find out*

about this by talking to the people who teach on it and people who train there including recent graduates. It is particularly important to speak to current trainees prior to applying. They give you the best sense of whether you can see yourself there. Nowadays it is easier to find things out by contacting people through Twitter and LinkedIn, for example. I would recommend to people that they should not hesitate to contact lots of people to hear about their experiences. It can all add to the picture. I would also encourage interested people not to shy away from having conversations with lecturers on the courses. Asking lots of questions is only going to give them a good impression!

In the final analysis, all of this research goes beyond a box-ticking exercise, however, and there may be variables that are intangible but important. "Trust your gut instinct", one of my colleagues says. "You may not know why you feel drawn to one course over another, but trust your intuition. It's like buying a house: buy the house you love, not the one that ticks all the boxes." So, armed with both your gut instincts and your grasp of all the practicalities, it is time to think about applying.

Applying to programmes

You will typically be making your application online, to include scanned and sent documents, although you may also submit elements of it via post or bring things with you on the day (for example, original degree certificates). Remember that even at this early stage, the programme team will be forming an impression of who you are and how you might manage the organisational challenges of a doctoral programme. If your application is rushed or messy, if it is incomplete or inaccurate (for example, if it has a personal statement that refers to another programme!), or if it appears to have been shoved in at the last minute, programme team members will already be wondering whether you are ready for this kind of course.

Despite the variations in counselling psychology programmes, their entry requirements are fairly consistent. Many of those requirements were mentioned in Chapter 3, but they are summarised below.

- Training programmes look for *evidence of academic ability to succeed on a doctoral programme*. They want you to have a 2:1 Honours undergraduate degree in psychology, or another kind of first degree plus a conversion course, conferring Graduate Basis for Chartership (GBC). If your undergraduate degree is a 2:2, courses will generally expect other evidence of your academic ability, such as successful completion of a Master's-level degree. Certain courses may ask you to submit a piece of critical writing or other coursework, and they will scrutinise your covering letter and/or personal statement for evidence of your ability to write well and clearly. Courses will likely require original degree certificates and will usually want to see full transcripts so that they can look at course content and your marks in different modules; you will need to contact the registry at your previous institution(s) for copies of these. Often courses require two letters of reference, and one of these should generally come from someone who can speak to your academic ability. Make sure to discuss your application with potential referees and check that it is all right to use them as a reference.

- *Graduate Basis for Chartership* (GBC) with the British Psychological Society, as discussed in Chapter 2. Courses will often want to see the letter from the BPS that verifies that you have this. If you are unable to locate the original letter, the BPS should be able to provide you with another. You may also be able to use your membership card.

- Training programmes want *evidence of the right kinds of relevant clinical experience* and generally require substantial experience in a helping role, preferably one-to-one counselling or mental health work. While other kinds of helping experiences may be considered relevant, courses usually want you to have gone beyond "befriending" type roles. They often specify approximately a year's experience, although this is sometimes difficult to define when experiences have been part-time. You will usually submit a CV with your application and/or fill out a form with details of your paid and unpaid relevant work experience. One of the two letters of reference that courses usually require should come from someone who is familiar with your clinical skills/work. Again, always ensure that you ask your referee ahead of time if it is all right for you to use them as a reference.

Programmes need *an indication of your ability to undertake research at doctoral level.* This is a bit of a challenge for them, as the only way to definitively prove doctoral mettle is to have completed a doctorate before! In the absence of that, the programme team will scrutinise the marks you have received for research modules and read any information they have about your experience with research, from you or from your referees. They will read through your personal statement to see if you seem aware of the importance of research within the training, and will also want to see indications that you have thought about what you might research at doctoral level. Some programmes ask you to submit a piece of past research with the application, or to produce a mini-proposal for a piece of doctoral research. Even if a given programme does not require you to submit a proposal, they are likely to appreciate your sending one. As one programme team member says, "It is great when [applicants] can demonstrate research-mindedness. This does not mean they need to have their doctoral research project sorted but that they can demonstrate interest in research and can talk about any previous research they have done coherently."

Programmes want to see *evidence of interpersonal skills and reflective abilities.* At written-application level, this is evidenced primarily through the personal statement that most programmes require; it is evaluated more deeply at the interview stage. Your letters of reference might also speak to this, particularly in the reference from the person who knows your clinical work.

If English is not your first language, courses will need to see *evidence of English proficiency.*

At some point in your training you will likely need to receive *clearance from the Disclosure and Barring Service* (DBS), formerly known as the CRB check, in order to see clients on clinical placement; in Scotland this is known as Disclosure Scotland (www.disclosurescotland.co.uk), in Northern Ireland AccessNI (www.nidirect.gov.uk). As a Graduate Member of the BPS, if you do not have a recent criminal records check, you can obtain one via the BPS, but if you do not have this on point of application (and many people do not), your course or one of your clinical placements will eventually facilitate it. Most programmes do not set your possession of an up-to-date check as a condition of application or admission.

- Many courses require you to have undertaken some kind of *formal counselling skills training*, although they may be flexible on the nature and the duration, and if you have not done it on point of application, this may be set as a condition of the offer of a place. All courses are likely to look more favourably upon your application if you have done this. Again, you will need to provide evidence of completion.

The criteria above are the standard baseline requirements for entry to counselling psychology programmes, and typically the admissions department scrutinises these initially to determine your face-value suitability for the course before passing your application to the programme team. If an application falls short on one or more of the above criteria, it may not make it to interview stage, and the admissions department or the programme team can give you information about why your application for interview was rejected. In practice, there is some flexibility; if you fall a bit short on a particular criterion, but other aspects of your application are quite strong, the programme may be curious enough about your potential to still call you in for an interview. Think carefully about taking this as an open license to "try your luck" if you clearly do not meet more than one admission criterion, however, not only because courses are competitive, but because meeting these criteria is an indication of readiness and suitability, and ready and suitable are two things you definitely want to be. Again, typically the admissions department undertakes an initial scrutiny of applications, ensuring that they meet the basic requirements. Applications that pass muster are then passed the course team, who determine who will be invited for interview.

Interviewing for a place

If you have made it to the interview stage, your written application has ticked all or most of the baseline criteria, but interview panels are looking for the more intangible aspects of your suitability for the programme. One trainer in counselling psychology sums it up this way:

> For programme teams . . . the role of professional gate-keeping begins here. Can we see this person as a member of the profession

of counselling psychology? . . . Do their personal characteristics demonstrate a commitment to the ethos of the counselling psychology profession? Does this person have the capability of developing into a counselling psychologist? Would I feel comfortable with this person as my therapist?

(Galbraith, 2016, p. 75)

What Galbraith is describing here has to do with the sometimes difficult-to-pin-down dimension of "personal suitability", in other words, whether the person seems to fit with the values and qualities of the profession that were outlined in Chapter 2. Beyond values, however, there is what one of my colleagues refers to as the "likeability factor". Clients entering therapy need to feel able to disclose, to make themselves vulnerable, and to do difficult psychotherapeutic work. If the personality or demeanour of a therapist does not foster feelings of safety, comfort and trust, it will be extremely difficult to form a working relationship. Because such impressions can be subjective and charged by individuals' personal reactions, applicants are usually evaluated by multiple individuals on the programme team, across multiple situations: question-and-answer sessions within informational presentations; individual interview(s); therapeutic role plays; group exercises or interactions; and/or written exercises. Applicants are often surprised by the degree to which personal suitability and personal experiences are considered in the interview process. Presented below are a variety of perspectives on this aspect of the interview process, from both trainers and trainees.

> **Nearly-qualified trainee counselling psychologist:** *My essay for the application was quite academic (I hadn't ever written a reflective essay before) and they asked me lots of questions about myself and my own process. It was a bit anxiety-provoking. I didn't think it was going to be so personal. I think they asked how my wish to train existentially related to my personal experience, and I can't remember what I responded, but I think I probably made quite an intellectual argument about positivism versus human exploration. I don't think I was really in touch with what this meant for me personally, and I think it had to do with some processes that I hadn't really acknowledged until later, when I started therapy.*

Programme team member: *When I was applying for training, my guesses about what they were looking for were probably wrong. In the group exercises I was naïve and took the discussion points at face value, not realising that the observation did not really concern* what *we were saying in the groups but* how *we were interacting with each other.*

Programme team member: *When I interview candidates now, I like to see that they are reflective, aware of their own issues, self-critical, willing to learn, open to other people's views, and non-defensive. If people have experienced mental health difficulties themselves, I like to see that they are open about it, neither avoidant and defensive, nor obsessive and preoccupied with it. This means they probably will have done some therapy and can reflect on their past in a balanced way.*

Programme team member: *Emotional honesty is really important, which involves the willingness to share your emotions with your fellow students and to explore those emotions with yourself. It's about the courage to be vulnerable.*

Multiple programme team members have emphasised to me that it is important for candidates to be able to explain why they want to train in counselling psychology in particular, and applicants are very likely to encounter questions that are designed to tap into (a) whether they understand what counselling psychology is, and (b) whether they have a clear sense of why it feels right for them. As the previous chapter emphasised, perhaps nothing annoys programme teams more than someone who applies to train without understanding the field or why they want to study it!

The chapter thus far has focused on university-based training programmes, but this route to qualification is not right for everyone's circumstances, so read on to consider the alternative.

Enrolling on the BPS Qualification in Counselling Psychology (QCoP)

While there are no significant differences between the taught route and the QCoP in the competencies and standards that must ultimately be achieved, some may argue that the similarities tail off from there. QCoP's alternative name, the "independent route", accurately captures its feel. If you pursue the QCoP, you will be undertaking a far more autonomous, self-driven way of reaching qualification as a counselling psychologist.

The process of enrolling on QCoP in some ways is a mirror image to the process of applying to the taught route. For trainees on the taught route, having been accepted onto a programme on the basis of their personal suitability and their meeting of certain criteria, they register on their programme first, and sort out their clinical supervision and placement situations second. On the QCoP, candidates identify a willing Coordinating Supervisor (CS) first (more on this later), and together with them they plan everything about their training – how they will gain their theoretical knowledge, what their placements will be, who will supervise their clinical work, what their research will be, and who will provide their personal therapy – and then submit all of this *as part of* their enrolment application for the QCoP. Upon application for enrolment, they submit a fully developed Plan of Training, approved by their CS; they may also make an application for Accreditation of Existing Competency (AEC). If the Registrar of the QCoP also approves the Plan of Training and other documentation, the candidate is enrolled and is free to proceed with their plan.

This system forces the candidate to be acutely conscious of qualification criteria, to be proactive in developing a strategy to meet these, and to own their training experience to a greater extent than on the course route. To some extent the flexibility and choice is similar to that on training courses – trainees on both routes choose their personal therapists, their placements, and often their clinical supervisors (when these are not provided on placement) – but on the QCoP the candidate also assumes responsibility for deciding where and how their core therapy training and working-model therapy training will take place.

In the last subsection, we looked at a variety of factors to ponder when considering the course route: location, structure, financial commitment, and content. With the QCoP, of course, *location* is incredibly flexible. You will need to do a postgraduate-level course-based core therapy training somewhere, which should involve 300–400 hours of contact on the course as well as supervised clinical practice, but this could take place anywhere that such courses exist. The same goes for your additional therapy training (for the "working knowledge" model(s)). The Coordinating Supervisors who approve and oversee your training are scattered throughout the UK, and they may or may not live near you. Placements can be arranged anywhere, as long as the placement meets QCoP criteria. In terms of *structure* and *content*, while you must plan and follow a training structure containing the kind of content that will help you meet the required competencies and standards, the precise way in which you configure your training is decided amongst you, your Coordinating Supervisor and the QCoP Registrar, and it will be significantly affected by the nature and extent of your existing experience and competencies.

The *financial commitment* on the QCoP is relatively low when compared to the course route. At the time of writing, the 2016 fees for the QCoP (which can be paid in various instalment schemes, spread over one to five years) was just over £11,100, and current fees are available on the BPS website. As with the course route, however, the fee for the actual QCoP is just the beginning of the story. The financial commitment for QCoP route to qualification is summarised in Table 4.2. As you will see, the cost calculation is a bit different than the one given above.

The person in Table 4.2 is not applying for any Accreditation of Existing Competence (AEC), and has already agreed fees with her CS, her external Placement Supervisor, her Research Supervisor, and her personal therapist. She is planning on circumventing any fee increases by paying in instalments over one year only.

As with the taught route, additional costs will likely be involved, to include: professional liability insurance, if your placement's insurance does not cover you; membership of the BPS and the Division of Counselling Psychology, charged at the trainee rate; Disclosure and Barring Service (DBS) checks, if this is not provided by your placement; and any books or other training materials you need or want to purchase. Wherever you live, even if you do not have physical access to a university library or to the BPS library Senate House, as a QCoP candidate you will have free online access to the Senate House library and to academic journals for the duration of your enrolment.

As you will see, even in Table 4.2, which involves someone who is not applying for AECs, the QCoP can cut the cost of training, particularly given that one can "shop around" for core therapy and additional therapy training or gain credit for existing qualifications and experiences through applying for AECs. For example, if someone had already undertaken a Master's degree that met the requirement for core therapy training; had already done 20 hours of personal therapy; had a Plan

Table 4.2 Calculating the cost of the QCoP

Expense	Amount	Notes
Fee for QCoP registration (2016)	£11,104 – pay within one year	The registration fee can be paid in instalments interest-free over 1–5 years; however, the fee can change annually, so you may pay more if you spread amount over a longer period.
Fee for regular meetings with/oversight by Coordinating Supervisor (CS)	£600 for each year, with three years on my Plan of Training – £600 × 3 = **£1,800**	A CS is likely to charge between £40 and £80 per hour, although some may be outside this range. You should assume between £400 and £800 for each year. Don't forget to multiply this by the number of years on your Plan of Training, and build in some margin. Negotiate fees and number of annual meetings with CS; check Candidate Handbook for minimum requirements. CS could charge per meeting or a flat rate annually.
Placement supervision, external to clinical placement	Given amount of supervision already provided internally on agreed clinical placement, I will need 40 hours of additional placement supervision. Supervisor X charges £60 per hour. 40 × £60 = **£2,400**	Practice supervisors external to clinical placements are likely to charge between £40 and £80 per hour, although some may be outside this range. It is wise to maximise any free supervision available on clinical placement(s). For 450 clinical hours you would need approximately 57 hours of clinical supervision over the course of your training.

(continued)

Table 4.2 *(continued)*

Expense	Amount	Notes
Research supervision	Supervisor Y and I have decided 20 hours will likely be needed – Supervisor Y charges £55 per hour. **20 × £55 = £1,100**	Research supervision is also likely to be between £40 and £80, although some will charge outside of this range. It can be difficult to work out how much research supervision you will need, so try to build in some level of margin. Those who have done at least a Master's level piece of research already may apply for AEC and will thus need very little, if anything, in the way of research supervision.
Personal therapy	My therapist charges £50 per hour. **40 × £50 = £2,000**	There are 40 hours required for the QCoP, and if you have had personal therapy in the past, you can claim AECs. Again, fees tend to range between £40 and £80.
Two-year core therapy training (existential) at Programme A – Master's in Psychotherapy and Counselling	**£8,000**	This is expected to consist of a professional training in one model of psychotherapy, comprising 300–400 course contact hours with 100 appropriately supervised client hours.
Additional therapy training (psychodynamic) at Programme B – Postgraduate Diploma in Psychodynamic Psychotherapeutic Counselling	£3,710	This is expected to consist of at least 150 course contact hours.
Total estimated costs	**£30,114**	

of Training lasting for two years rather than three; and had already undertaken a suitable piece of research, the costs of that person's QCoP training would amount to only £19,414. Compared to most course routes, the QCoP is relatively open and flexible with respect to crediting AECs, and this makes a significant difference.

All of the information about enrolment on the QCoP can be found on the "Society Qualifications" section of the BPS website, www.bps.org. uk. Good first steps include reviewing all the documents found there – to include the handbooks, regulations, and guidance documents – and hooking into one of the QCoP Registrar's regular telephone clinics. The Qualifications Team are also available to answer questions, and there is a member of that team dedicated to the QCoP; their contact is also on the BPS website. The website also contains information on how to find approved Coordinating Supervisors, which is the next step to take once you are fairly certain you wish to enrol. All Coordinating Supervisors for the QCoP must undergo formal training and regular continuing professional development to maintain their accreditation. Once you find someone, your CS will guide you through the enrolment process.

Even if the flexibility and potentially lower cost of the QCoP (depending on how you arrange it) are appealing, you may wonder how it *feels* relative to the course route. The next sections consider life as a taught-route candidate versus life as a QCoP trainee. Everyone's experiences and preferences are different, but the accounts in the next section(s) provide a bit of an indication.

Life as a trainee

Life as a taught-route counselling psychology trainee

Ask a counselling psychology trainee what their life is like, and a handful of themes crop up again and again. On one hand, you will hear about stimulation, challenge, excitement, and fulfilment. On the other, you will hear about a lot of stress and anxiety, much of it unanticipated. While everyone's experience is unique, a few key aspects of course training are highlighted here. Acknowledgement of the more stressful elements is not intended to intimidate you, or put you off of the idea of training; it is included to help you to be realistic about what this kind of experience may be like, and to go into it with your eyes open.

If there is one thing that you will need to be ready for, it is the sensation of being on what a colleague of mine calls, "the train that doesn't stop". Once you board you will find that it is difficult to disembark and catch your breath! This unstoppable train feeling is related to the fact that most (although not all) counselling psychology doctorates are cohort-based trainings. This has its joys and sorrows, as we will see.

The majority of counselling psychology training programmes have one or two intakes of trainees per year, depending on the resources and size of the programme. In this structure, the cohort moves through their training as a group, spending most of their time with one another. As you can imagine, cohorts often become quite cohesive on training courses such as this, as they are far more than just people sitting together in lectures. They interact and work together closely in seminars, sometimes collaborating on group projects; they engage in dyad or triad work when developing their clinical skills, in exercises that may involve real-life material; they support one another through the various experiences of training; and they spend virtually all of their classroom time together over three to four years. The relationships that develop here can be extraordinarily strong, as described in the quote below.

> **Early-career qualified counselling psychologist:** *A nice thing about being on a course was being part of a cohort of trainees. I still see many of them and am in contact with many others I met during my training. We feel not like friends and not like colleagues, but like siblings. Despite all our differences, there is an enduring bond between us.*

In their closeness, members of a given cohort may utilise each other quite extensively. When asked how trainees can get the support they need, one nearly-qualified trainee emphasises the importance of the cohort:

> **Nearly-qualified trainee counselling psychologist:** *No one outside your cohort will understand what you're going through – except counselling psychologist trainees from other courses you meet on placement. Be open. Ask for help. Don't just emotionally support each other, work together academically too, share essays and ideas. Try and be a learning community.*

One of the quotes above compares members of a cohort to siblings, and as with siblings, interpersonal dynamics within a cohort may not always be comfortable or smooth. The nature of the profession means that cohort members tend to come from vastly diverse backgrounds. It could be argued this actually lends an additional and valuable dimension to counselling psychology training, as one first-year trainee describes:

> **First-year trainee counselling psychologist:** *I love the diversity of my year group. I love the professions everybody's come from, and I think that the course, although it has these criteria for getting in, you look around our eclectic bunch, and it's kind of like wow, we're all learning the same stuff, bringing these things . . . That's a challenge and a blessing. It's a challenge in that you do have to be inclusive, but it's brilliant because it can include you too, whoever you are.*

Cohorts of trainees on a counselling psychology doctorate will usually proceed along a fixed programme of modules in a particular order, with each module likely to be offered just once a year, and this has significant implications. Here comes the flip side of being attached to a particular group of trainees. If you were to struggle with one or more modules, your progression onto the next stage might be affected; depending on your programme's regulations, you *may* be able to retake a failed module the next time it runs, but that might not be until the following year. You might also need to take time out from the programme for personal reasons. In either case, whenever you push the pause button – or have it pushed for you – you will inevitably fall behind while the rest of your original cohort forges ahead. Concerns about losing their place within their "trainee family" provide a powerful incentive for many trainees to stay on that train no matter what.

Despite their intent and desire to stick to the plan, many trainees encounter significant challenges, often unexpected. Some of these have to do with academic work, either the *amount* of academic work, or the *standard* of work expected. As covered in the previous chapter, there is a significant jump between undergraduate- and Master's-level work and the doctorate, and this may prove particularly flummoxing for trainees who have been out of the academic setting for a while and/or who do not have English as a first language. The following accounts are typical narratives from counselling psychology trainees about the academic challenges they encountered on their training programmes.

> **First-year trainee counselling psychologist:** *I couldn't get my head around how to write an essay with an original argument and yet substantiate it with what's already there, and I didn't realise that so much reading would go into one 3,000-word essay!*

> **Second-year trainee counselling psychologist:** *When I started the course, I had done my undergrad 10 years ago, and it was straight onto this doctorate. From the perspective of academic writing, I found that really difficult. I had done writing for my work, so I felt comfortable-ish with the structure and stuff, but in terms of criticality and having the confidence to compare and pull apart other people's work . . . I was like, "that's gospel! . . . you can't touch that!"*

> **Third-year trainee counselling psychologist:** *A struggle most of my classmates and I came across was the intensity of the course and the pressure we felt from lecturers. I assumed that it would carry on at a similar pace as my Master's, but the requirements for the academic side of it were overwhelming for me. I found it particularly difficult to write big assignments in a foreign language to such a high standard. Also the pressure from lecturers and tutors to "get it right otherwise it's a failure" left me feeling that I couldn't do it! I had great support in friends who proofread my work and helped me with my English. I was also able to do the course part-time in second year, as I realised that pace does suit me better. I learned to reflect more deeply and to take care of myself better.*

> **Nearly-qualified trainee counselling psychologist:** *I'd been warned that it would be hard work. Once I was accepted onto the course, I looked at the timetable and syllabus, and thought, "well, that's a lot of essays, but I've been working and studying for years – I'll be fine". I couldn't have been more wrong. The academic pressure was brutal.*

Academic requirements, however, are only one strand. The core feature of a practitioner doctorate in counselling psychology is its multifaceted nature. During training, whichever course you choose, you will be undertaking the following:

- *Academic*: Completing over 500 academic credit hours, with associated reading and preparation of coursework.

- *Clinical*: Undertaking at least 450 direct hours with clients; completing additional associated placement-related hours; and typically obtaining somewhere between 57 and 75 hours of clinical supervision, dependent on the requirements of the course.

- *Research*: Reviewing literature, developing proposal(s), going through ethics approval processes, recruiting participants, analysing data, writing up, having vivas and/or readying work for publication.

- *Personal development*: Undertaking personal therapy as a requirement (the various programmes differ widely and may stipulate anywhere from 40 to 160 hours), keeping self-development journals, attending personal and professional development groups.

So, as they trundle along on the train that does not stop, trainees are engaged in an elaborate juggling act. Keeping coursework, placements, research, supervision, and personal therapy going simultaneously is no mean feat, and as many of the following testimonials illustrate, this can exact a considerable personal toll. Once again, I feel poised on the edge between honesty and nondisclosure, and find myself wondering what will happen if I let you in on just how hard this can be! I ask myself whether it will it discourage people from training. Fortunately, nearly every trainee and qualified counselling psychologist who experiences these challenges also reaps rewards.

Nearly-qualified trainee counselling psychologist: *It will be harder than you think, in terms of time, effort and money, and especially, emotion. Warn your partner, family, friends, anyone involved with you, that, on the rare occasions they see you in the next few years, you will be a wreck. Tell them not to expect too much from you. Get ready to disappoint them. The joys are in the learning – academic and personal – and in clinical work. This has been incredibly hard, but I've never regretted it.*

Nearly-qualified trainee counselling psychologist: *Question – how do you become a counselling psychologist? Answer – you can do it the hard way, or you can do it the hard way.*

Nearly-qualified trainee counselling psychologist: *The academic pressure was brutal, the personal challenges were brutal, the lack of money was brutal, the amount of time I spent travelling between placements struggling to get my hours was brutal. On top of that, for five or six hours a week I had to put myself aside and learn how to be with a client. It was – well, hard work doesn't describe it. What kept me going through the pain was that I was constantly being stretched, and challenged, and there were moments of enormous excitement and joy at what, and how much, I was learning.*

Early-career qualified counselling psychologist: *Looking back, I would say it was quite tough. I had to juggle family and training, and my marriage broke down six months before I graduated – relationship breakdowns are very common during training. I underestimated how much the training changed me, and that my partner could not cope with this. Maybe I would not have gone into the training, had I known this beforehand. Yet I cannot say I have regrets, as I feel passionate about the profession, and I feel that the training may have only brought to the surface what was unworkable in the relationship anyway.*

Early-career qualified counselling psychologist: *While managing the demands of research and practice on the training, undergoing one's own therapy is an additional factor that can rock the boat. Having said all this, I also loved my training. It was a journey of discovery, whether this concerned learning about clients, theories, myself, and research areas, and it felt the right thing to do for me, with all its challenges.*

Nearly-qualified trainee counselling psychologist: *I would advise future trainees to consider the impact the course has on all aspects of your life. My course certainly emphasises self-reflection, and awareness of the interaction of personal and professional life, and I was particularly tested during my time on the course. The important thing is: life happens. Life still goes on around you when you're focusing on supporting clients, and fulfilling course needs of hours, essays, lecture input. Don't be fooled: this is an intense course. To become a counselling psychologist is to develop an identity through your training and experiences, and this identity does not leave you when you go home.*

This can be positive and fulfilling, but it can also be painful and confusing, and force you to face parts of you that you may not want to face, just as we ask our clients to do. Be careful to maintain boundaries and explain to friends and family that you are not able to counsel them in times of need, and that you still have needs from them of love and support, often even more so on your journey as a trainee. Knowing how to help others does not always mean you can help yourself. Becoming a counselling psychologist is an intense, painful, wonderful, insightful, and most of all a transformational experience; but also one I would not change for the world.

Several of the accounts above reference the clinical-placements element of training, which is clearly a major component of training, and about which more will be said in the next chapter. Before we get to that, however, it is worth saying a few words about the rather different experience of being an independent-route QCoP trainee.

Life as an independent-route counselling psychology trainee

The experience of QCoP converges with that of the taught route in some places, and diverges with it in others. Certainly, the standards and competencies one must demonstrate at the end of training are exactly the same, although the means by which they are achieved and shown often differs. In the section above, I outline the various strands of taught-route training, and now I go through them again, with some notes about how they play out differently as a candidate on the QCoP.

- *Academic*: The QCoP is a BPS qualification rather than an academic degree, so instead of accumulating academic credits, candidates complete Documentary Evidence Units (DEUs) and submit Assessment Units (AUs) to evidence their learning, which are marked by a team of assessors and moderated by the chief assessor and an examination board. Two of those DEUs do, however, involve taking psychotherapy courses to learn the candidate's chosen core and working model(s) of psychotherapy; if candidates already have these under their belts, they can get Accreditation of Existing Competence (AEC).

QCoP candidates will do a significant amount of coursework while doing the Qualification, and this coursework is assessed in the same way as on a taught route. A team of QCoP assessors, who have been trained to do the job, mark candidates' work, overseen by a chief assessor. The QCoP Examination Board is the final-sign off, similarly to university examination boards, and the QCoP has an external examiner, as courses do. As with the course route, candidates need to do substantial reading to support their learning.

- *Clinical*: Placements are planned and arranged before candidates embark on the Qualification, and their Plan of Training will be expected as part of the enrolment process. Once placements are established, the experience of clinical placements on the QCoP is more or less indistinguishable from being on the course route. The supervision hour to clinical hour ratio is 1:8, although most candidates do more than 57 supervision hours. Because candidates are not being taught by counselling psychologists on a course, they may struggle more with developing a true "counselling psychology identity" – because of this, the QCoP requires Coordinating Supervisors to be chartered by the BPS and HCPC-Registered Counselling Psychologists. While some placement supervisors may have other relevant accreditations, all candidates must have placement supervision from a counselling psychologist for the majority of their training; since availability of counselling psychologists varies geographically, this input may vary.

- *Research*: Research will most likely be undertaken as part of a relevant Master's, either one undertaken in the past, or one embarked upon as part of the QCoP. Interestingly, even though the QCoP overall is considered to be at doctoral level, the research one needs to have undertaken on the QCoP need only be at M-level. (Again, a significant number of other units are marked at doctoral level, and there is no AEC available for these units.) An additional reflective essay on the relevance of the research to counselling psychology practice may be required.

- *Personal development*: The QCoP currently requires a minimum of 40 hours of personal therapy, for which a candidate may claim AECs. This is a considerable difference from taught routes, which may require anything between 40 and 160 hours, but which will also usually require that personal therapy to be undertaken concurrent with the training programme.

What immediately strikes one about QCoP is the difference from a highly structured, cohort-based training. Together with their Coordinating Supervisor, the QCoP candidate plots an individualised course; undertakes it at a pace and in an order that best suits them; and navigates it largely alone. Without question, this pulls on a different set of skills, and will not suit all personalities – even for more naturally solitary and self-driven types, it is not all roses. The qualified counselling psychologist below describes her own experience of a life on the Qualification.

Case study of a qualified counselling psychologist, trained on QCoP: *I did my psychology Master's in Poland, moved to UK after that, and took time to settle. For a while, I didn't know what to do. A postgraduate diploma in counselling caught my eye, as I wanted to be a therapist working with clients. I did not realise, however, that it was only focused on the person-centred approach, and in time I found this quite limiting in my work with clients. I wanted to join my psychology degree and also expand to other ways of working. I came across counselling psychology, which seemed more what I was looking for in terms of including my own personal reflecting and personal therapy. My friend was doing an independent route in counselling psychology, so I decided to enrol as well. I was surprised how much of my experience I could use as Accreditation of Existing Competency.*

It was a lonely and difficult route – but I do well working on my own. People usually find their support groups, either though work or the courses they take. I was in the northwest of England, and we created the Northwest Division of Counselling Psychology (DCoP) branch for people to connect, link, and support each other. In that branch we have quite a few independent-route trainees at the moment.

I found it quite difficult to have been doing the independent route and then to join a course for my top-up doctorate. The course has its culture, and I found it really hard to get into this culture, which had an impact on how I did my assessments and how they were marked. Although the issues of being different are not new to me, as a Polish-born person in the UK, I felt I did not fit in on the course, which was already established.

Part of my experience was about feeling like I was working the whole time – first in my normal job, and then evenings, weekends and holidays

doing the training. To be honest, it got worse I went further into train-
ing! Having a part-time job and doing the training seem to fit well, but
doing a full-time job and the training was really hard.

You will note several things about this account. First, this QCoP candidate was able to *work while she was undertaking the training.* The relatively structured, inflexible, train-not-stopping nature of many taught routes – some of which do not even allow for the possibility of completing some parts of the course on a part-time basis – will certainly make full-time work virtually impossible, and will challenge attempts at part-time work as well. For this reason, some experience the QCoP as more financially achievable.

Second, this practitioner highlights her ability, on the QCoP, to *use much of her prior experience towards AECs.* Again, many taught routes do not permit much in the way of accreditation of prior learning. On the flip side, however, this practitioner elected for personal and employability reasons to undertake a top-up doctorate, since the QCoP itself does not result in a doctorate, despite being doctoral level. As she describes, this was a considerable culture shock after working independently on her training for some time.

Third, she notes the *relative loneliness/autonomy of undertaking the QCoP* and highlights the need to find ways of combatting this. Time and logistics permitting, many QCoP candidates strive to find ways of connecting with other trainees, whether those trainees are independent candidates or not. Trainee-focused BPS events, social media platforms such as the counselling psychology Facebook page, and attendance at conferences – useful points of contact for any trainee – may be even more useful for the trainee pursuing QCoP. QCoP trainees also all have access to a web forum set up specifically for them.

Finding clinical placements

Although there are many academic elements, counselling psychology training is primarily a *professional* one. You learn theory with the primary aim of translating it into practice, and the research you undertake will benefit and inform professional psychologists. Unsurprisingly, therefore, your clinical placements constitute a huge percentage of your learning.

QCoP candidates cannot even enrol without already-secured placements, but on the taught route, the need to secure placement(s) as swiftly as possible can be a source of considerable anxiety during the first year in particular. There are, however, many ways that you can prevent this from being overly stressful.

As emphasised earlier in this book, counselling psychology differs from some of the other branches of applied psychology in that its training courses do not require specific, pre-determined types of placements. While most programmes have placement coordinator(s) or placement administrator(s) that can assist, and while programmes usually maintain large databases of potential placements, not all of them have relationships or set arrangements with particular placement providers. To be on the safe side, a counselling psychology trainee should plan to be relatively self-driven during the placement acquisition process. What can you do to help your cause?

First, *network early and often.* Even before you begin your training – in fact, before you apply – start nurturing your relationships with the practitioners you encounter. It goes without saying that you should build relationships with the professionals that you meet while undertaking counselling work experience, but you can network further by joining the counselling psychology's "discourse community" to make even more connections. Join the Division of Counselling Psychology group on Facebook, and/or follow @dcopuk on Twitter. Before you even join a programme, attend the Division of Counselling Psychology annual conference, and/or the main BPS conference. Have discussions with the people you meet, tell them about your plans to train, collect their details, and follow up with email contact afterwards. "Definitely get on with it early", one trainee told me, "because no one replies for ages and you panic! Then they all come in at once three months later on." Meeting the required therapy hours at the end of the year is not the only reason why trainees panic; not having a clinical placement earlier in the year can also interfere with your ability to complete clinically-based coursework, such as process reports and case studies. So get out and start talking with people!

Second, *do advance research* on the psychological services in your locality, and around the locality where you arc training/hope to train. If a particular placement is not on a programme's list, it will generally be approved by your course if it meets the criteria for a training placement. "I started looking for placements that were not on the list and managed to find an organisation quite quickly that offered me a placement", says one nearly-qualified trainee. "After discussing [how it met the requirements] with my tutor, I was able to start practising immediately. I found two out of my four placements on my own, and now other students are there on placement as well." This leads us naturally into the third tip.

Third, once you are on a training programme, *get help through trainees on the cohort(s) above you*. The more experienced trainees already established in placements will not feel themselves to be in competition with you and will remember the difficulty and anxiety of securing placements, and are hence often very willing to help. In addition, managers and supervisors at those placements will be familiar with your programme and its procedures. If it has not already been compiled, ask your placement tutor or placements coordinator for a "shortlist" of those services that have provided placements to trainees on your programme over the last few years – this usually represents a substantial edit of what may be an overwhelmingly large placements database.

Fourth, make sure that you are *utilising all the resources available* to you. Read up on finding clinical placements (Bor & Watts, 2017; Lawrence, 2016). If you are applying to lots of places but not getting much joy, and you are on the taught route at a university, there will usually be individuals in central services (e.g., careers office, academic skills) that can help with your CV, your cover letters, and your interviewing skills. You may also be able to consult your personal tutor, and/or your placements tutor/coordinator, to ask how you can improve your chances. One first-year trainee who had recently availed herself of the careers office at her university endorsed this heartily, pointing out that a CV rewrite might be in order if you have not applied for clinical placements before. "We arrive with varied and complicated backgrounds", she said. "Those need to be translated to saleable skills on a CV for placement applications."

Finally, while it can be tempting to take the first placements you are offered, do try to *be strategic* about your future employability. If you know where you would like to end up, you can get quite specific about this. One nearly-qualified trainee has the following advice: "Look at where the jobs are – sign up to NHS jobs – and plan accordingly. If you can, plan it so that you cover different areas. One person I know started in a school, then worked in an adult counselling charity, and finally took a placement in a service for older adults, nicely covering a lifespan spectrum. Others took specialist placements like substance misuse or learning disabilities. If you plan your placements carefully, you can develop a specialism."

One of my own counselling psychology trainees compiled the following "top tips" on securing clinical placements. As she was in the first year at the time of putting this list together, the experience of finding placements was fresh in her mind.

First-year counselling psychology trainee – top tips

- *Acquiring a placement does not happen overnight; I underestimated the time it takes to apply, interview, complete paperwork, and so forth. It's a long and often slow process. I had instances of applying to placements in October and not being offered an interview until the New Year. So don't panic if everything is taking slightly longer than you thought.*

- *Apply anyway! I came across numerous placements specifying that only second- or third-years need apply. But for those I really liked the look of I applied anyway. You 100% know that you won't be offered a placement if you haven't even applied. It turns out that both of my current placements (Mind and NHS Psychosis) originally posted for second-years. Sometimes being an optimist pays off!*

- *Interviews are a two way process – they're an opportunity for you ask questions too. If an organisation is coming across as disorganised and unprofessional, it might be worth asking yourself, "Will I feel supported here? Is this going to be a good learning environment?"*

- *Sell yourself and your course. It pays off to read around the organisation you are applying for, current projects, their therapeutic models, and so forth, but don't neglect what being on your current course can offer a placement. My course emphasises the existential model, and whilst I am still early on in my training both my placements expressed an interest in having someone on the team who will be developing within this paradigm.*

- *Be honest. Your interviewers will know your stage of training and will not expect you to know everything. What became very apparent within my interviews is that the emphasis was placed on my thought processes rather than being able to directly relate to every scenario-based question. For example, when I was asked, "Have you been in X situation, and how did you handle it?" my response was centred around what I would do.*

- *Call, don't email. Emails get lost and put off, but it's harder to ignore a ringing phone. You feel slightly like a stalker, but I've found it is a great way of getting answers to questions and moving through paperwork quickly. It also provides an opportunity to build rapport with whomever answers the phone, which could be key to getting someone to look at your CV.*

As so many accounts in this chapter make clear, whatever training route you are taking to qualification, your path will be replete with both joys and challenges. You can think of this period as the "Novice Student" phase (Rønnestad & Skovholt, 2012), and you will spend much of your time making sense of all of the information being thrown at you. It is the first, and perhaps the steepest, ascent on what will be a long learning curve. Most counselling psychology students wrestle initially with the various intellectual, practical, and emotional tasks of training. The theory, the uncertainty and self-doubt around one's ability to apply that theory in practice, the panic over acquiring placements, the questions about whether you can hack it – these are all par for the course. By the middle of the second year or so, you will be moving into the "Advanced Student" phase and beginning to anticipate or even experience the "Novice Professional" phase (ibid.). The next chapter will consider how you can make the most of the latter part of your training, and how you can set yourself up well for the early post-qualification period.

5 Starting out

This chapter gives you a sense of what you can do both before and after qualification to get the best possible start in professional life as a counselling psychologist. If you are reading this book as an A-level or undergraduate psychology student, think of it as a useful resource for learning more about what it is like to move from training to working life, and for planning ahead. If you are using this book as someone who is already a trainee counselling psychologist, the chapter may be of more immediate use to you in positioning yourself well, and in service of maximum employability.

If one day you find yourself ensconced in practice as a counselling psychologist, do not expect to look back and be able to clearly identify the moment at which your career actually launched. The start of professional life is not a precisely defined point, something that occurs instantaneously when all coursework is finished, when the doctoral examiners offer their congratulations, when the degree certificate is on the wall or when the HCPC registration card arrives in the post.

One of the reasons that the transition between trainee and professional life is diffuse is that the experience of professionalisation occurs gradually rather than in stages. The experience and knowledge gained over the years of early training means that latter-stage trainees often feel like confident quasi-professionals with skills and agency. At the same time, "the professional self is still fragile" (Rønnestad & Skovholt, 2012, p. 72), and there may be considerable oscillation between competence and insecurity. Conscious of the fact that qualification is approaching, trainees undertake more deliberate reflection on the professional choices they are making, and take greater ownership of their career trajectory. Some of the key developmental tasks of the novice professional phase – to include developing an identification with and commitment to the field, and exploring and defining one's professional role – start well before qualification as a counselling psychologist.

There are other reasons why the transition between training and post-qualified life feels a bit messy or indistinct. One or more training placements may morph into a "proper job", blurring the boundary between trainee and qualified professional. Certain factors can delay registration and chartership, which will be discussed later in this chapter; these may limit job choices at or, at worst, leave a person in employability limbo. Finally, both *feelings* of proficiency and competence and *actual* proficiency and competence can decline as well as increase after qualification.

The graph in Figure 5.1, adapted from Rosenberg (2014), gives you a sense of what can happen if you do not treat the time *after* qualification as a time for continued learning and accumulation of proficiencies. Line A illustrates a fantasy that some trainees may have, that is, that your formal counselling psychology training will give you all that you need to launch as a professional. What actually happens is more like Line B. You are perhaps less ready than you think you are, but your training will still have equipped you well for success, depending on what you do next. If you abandon your learning, mentorship and close

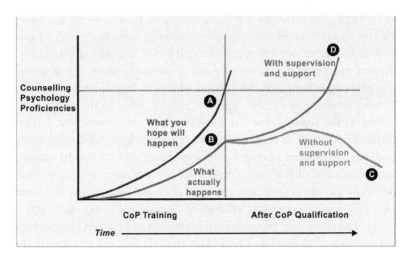

Figure 5.1   Maintenance of competencies after training

Adapted from Rosenberg, M. (2014). Why support after training is important [Internet Article]. Available on: http://learningsolutionsmag.com/articles/1348/ marc-my-words-the-training-to-competence-myth.

supervisory support too quickly after graduation, your proficiency level could actually go down rather than up, as illustrated by line C, perhaps without your even realising it. When post-qualification learning is reinforced and supported, however, your expertise and competence will only build, as in line D.

So, this chapter is designed to help you understand what is necessary to achieve another of the developmental tasks for the novice professional: "to succeed in the transformation from the dependency of graduate school to the independence that is expected, both from oneself and from others, after having completed professional training" (Rønnestad & Skovholt, 2012, p. 83). Because of the importance of the pre-qualification period for later success, a substantial portion of the chapter is given over to this phase.

Going the extra mile before you qualify

Just completing the baseline requirements to qualify and to register can occupy most of your time and energy. Trainees describe the overall work of juggling their multitudinous commitments and strands of training – reading, coursework, training placements, supervision, personal therapy, research – as being the most challenging thing about their training years. If you enter training, you are likely to have a similar experience. Once one is in the thick of it, it is hard to imagine doing anything "extra" over the course of the training. Those extras that are difficult to make time for, however, eventually make a person more employable on graduation than the average newly-minted C.Psychol. (Chartered Psychologist). Beyond employability considerations, doing these things will help you to become more "expert", to develop your identity as a counselling psychologist, and to feel a more integral part of the professional community that you are seeking to join.

The following account is from a trainee counselling psychologist who has taken an extremely proactive and strong approach to doing additional work off-course, which ultimately she doesn't really see as "extra" at all!

Case study of a first-year trainee counselling psychologist taking her learning "off course": *A professional doctorate in counselling psychology can be stressful and overwhelming. There is always too much* *to read and to write, too much to do and to think about. And the anxiety! Am I good enough? Will I pass the exam? Will I do what is expected of me . . . and what is expected of me anyway? There is little to hold on to, since every guideline, every handbook, and every instruction for an assessment has caveats and is accompanied by "yes, but" – precisely how you meet competencies and standards is up to you. All of this is in service of our chosen end: to be a practitioner who is aware of rather than molded by.*

To me, this entails going beyond the knowledge that the ivory halls of university can offer me. Since I started my training last year, I have attended workshops and seminars on Acceptance & Commitment Therapy (ACT) and Relational Frame Theory (RFT); I've been to the general BPS conference and to the Division of Counselling Psychology conference; and I've done teacher-training in autogenics, mindfulness-based stress reduction (MBSR) and mindfulness-based cognitive therapy (MBCT). Believe me, I fail exams like everyone else, get lower grades than I want, and struggle with the same fears that my peers do; however, I want to acquire more skills and connect to people who are at different places in their careers. I feel that it is important to see the course as one means to an end, though many means are needed to create the practitioner I want to be.

This approach is not only enriching this first-year trainee's experience in the moment, it is forward-thinking and will likely help her get a job upon qualification. Many of the things she highlights in her account are expanded upon in the sections below.

Plan to get extra training and support to supplement your core training

Over the course of your training, you may have identified a particular specialty that you want to develop, and there is no reason to wait until you qualify to augment your expertise. With an eye towards your future employability, keep abreast of what is happening in the marketplace – for example, a therapeutic approach that is gaining in popularity. Think about what kinds of extra training you can search out that might position you to take best advantage of emerging opportunities when you qualify.

Extra training and support can come from a number of different places, including the institution where you are undertaking your training if you are on a taught route; events sponsored by the Division of Counselling Psychology or the wider BPS, some of which are specifically aimed at trainees; continuing professional development (CPD) provided by other organisations; online courses and webinars; and training situated within your clinical placements. Whatever you undertake, ensure that you keep a record, as well as anything else (e.g., certificates) that will evidence your attendance. Even if your programme does not require it, create a table of the HCPC *Standards of Proficiency* and record any extra training against the various standards it has helped you meet. In a workshop with my third-year trainees recently, one particularly keen trainee who had attended a huge number of conferences confessed that she had not collected a single certificate of attendance along the way! Make an early habit of saving everything like this, and remember that it is useful for more reasons than just being able to evidence your proficiencies – every second year the HCPC chooses names at random and audits practitioner psychologists to ensure they are keeping up their continuing professional development.

Once you are qualified, there is no reason to rest on your laurels – keep on developing along trajectories that will make you a specialist in particular areas. The counselling psychologist below gives her own example of developing both in-training and post-training competencies and specialisms.

Case study of a mid-career (12 years) qualified counselling psychologist: *The placement that helped me to get a job was an eating disorders placement at the National Centre for Eating Disorders, working directly for someone who was a professional icon within the field. This experience later helped me to secure an adolescent job in Child and Adolescent Mental Health Services (CAMHS). I made sure that in my training I covered all the areas and did placements in learning disabilities, older adults, and enhanced primary care – you really have to get good placements in order to secure a job in the NHS. I became a community psychologist in a Sure Start, and I was then promoted into my current job in CAMHS as an adolescent specialist. I would tell trainees not to be put off and to get as much high quality NHS experience as possible while training, but I also really* *recommend post-qualification training. I am now a certified schema therapist for adults, adolescents and children (advanced), I have additional qualifications in Dialectical Behaviour Therapy (DBT), and I have done a lot of training in personality disorders to make complex adolescents my specialty.*

Whether you are still in training or post qualification, if you are a member of the BPS, you can use the "MyCPD" online planning and recording tool on the Professional Development Centre area of the BPS website to keep track of everything. That brings us on to the next tip.

Think about becoming involved in your professional organisation during training

Some training courses require you to be an in-training member of the Division of Counselling Psychology and others make this optional, but even those trainees who *are* members often are not aware of all of the perks of membership. As an in-training member you will be able to access conference bursaries, discounts on books, liability insurance deals, and the Senate House library in London. Benefits for trainee members are not the only consideration, however, and the greater your involvement whilst still a trainee, the more your future employability can be enhanced.

There are numerous ways of becoming involved with the BPS generally and with the Division of Counselling Psychology specifically, one of which is to be a trainee representative on the Divisional Committee. When I served on that committee, the trainee representative at the time accumulated a host of experiences and skills for his CV – for example, he organised trainee talks and other events, and collaborated with other members of the Division, such as the Training Lead and myself as Research Lead, on key projects affecting trainees. Furthermore, the contacts he made while on the committee resulted in his being contracted to contribute to a book chapter before he even graduated.

Another way of getting involved with the BPS and the Division is through conferences. At the time of writing, the Division of Counselling Psychology sponsors two ambassadors each year to represent counselling psychology at the main BPS conference; in this role, you not only strengthen your CV but also further develop your professional identity while promoting the field. The Conference Committee for the Division is also nearly always looking for trainee involvement, but even if you are not on that committee, you can volunteer to be a steward at the annual Division of Counselling Psychology conference, which means free attendance, being able to watch the presentations that you are overseeing, and hearing all of the keynote presentations once you have helped everyone to their places! You will need to keep an eye on the conference website and the Division of Counselling Psychology's regular e-Letter to stay in touch with opportunities as they arise.

Plan to publish early – and even often!

Candidates on traditional PhDs are no strangers to publishing work along the road to the doctorate, but within counselling psychology – perhaps because of the busy, multi-stranded nature of doing a professional doctorate – it seems to be relatively unusual for people to publish whilst still in training. Publishing your work early, however, is one of the best ways to stand out from the crowd of newly-qualified practitioners. If you apply for a job and your potential employers can access an article authored by you, they will have a much clearer sense of your skills as a thinker, practitioner, and/or researcher, and it may imbue you with greater "expert" status than the next applicant; furthermore, the initiative shown by early publication demonstrates a particular level of commitment to your profession. Finally, even if you have no intention of entering academia at this point, you never know where life will take you; many practitioners eventually include teaching in their repertoire. Not all teaching and training posts require publications, but there is no question that your chances of obtaining a faculty position will be reduced if you have none. Why limit your future opportunities?

If you think that you need to wait until you have substantially completed your doctoral research before trying your hand at publication, think again. You are studying and writing at a high level, and you are producing myriad types of coursework, including but not limited to your research. Virtually all counselling psychology trainees are required to undertake case studies, for example. If you have the appropriate informed consent from your clients – and I recommend using an informed consent form that covers a number of different eventualities – you potentially have the basis for a piece that could be published in a journal devoted to clinical case studies. All trainees also produce essays somewhere along the way. If you have produced an essay with a novel or original angle, or if you have put together a strong critical literature review in preparation for your doctoral research, what do you have to lose by attempting to get it published, in a journal that features a variety of different types of articles? While material produced for the purposes of coursework submission is almost never in publication-ready format, revamping it for a journal is less work than you might imagine, and your lecturer, personal tutor, or research supervisor may be willing to help you, particularly if second authorship is an incentive. Keep an eye out as well for competitions or other publication opportunities. At the time of writing, for example, the Division of Counselling Psychology awards a yearly prize for the best piece of (non-research) coursework authored by a trainee, which then yields you a publication in *Counselling Psychology Review*.

On the research side of things, if you produced a particularly spectacular undergraduate thesis or an excellent Master's dissertation, and you have not yet crafted it into a journal article, set aside some time to do that, getting support and utilising good guidance if this is new territory for you (e.g., Thomson & Kamler, 2012). Ideally you should voice your intent to publish articles based on your doctoral research to your supervisory team/your Director of Studies from your very first meeting with them – even if they are not pushing it with you – but if you do not do this in the beginning, it is never too late. The BPS has produced a policy statement on authorship and publication credit, which specifies that supervisors should be entitled to second authorship on any articles deriving from the research they supervise, and this should serve as an incentive to any supervisor who is also interested in advancing their own career!

Build in time and funding to engage in conferencing throughout your training

When I use the word "conferencing", I am referring to the whole range of possibilities. You can use conferences purely as learning and networking opportunities – do not forget the CPD certificate point made earlier – or you can present, in a number of different formats. Many conferences allow you to present work in progress, particularly for a poster.

If your research is at an advanced stage, or if you have a particular area of expertise, you have even more conferencing options. Let's say that you have become quite the expert in your research methodology over the course of your doctorate. In that case, consider submitting an abstract for a workshop to spread your knowledge to others. If other trainees in your cohort or programme are undertaking research in a similar topic area, band together to form a symposium, or go it alone and submit an abstract for an individual paper. Most conferences require you to have substantially completed your research (e.g., data collected and analysed) before they will accept your work for an individual paper or component of a symposium.

It goes without saying that the more conferences you attend, the more people in the field you will get to know. Because counselling psychologists are employed in all sorts of working contexts, do not limit yourself to the counselling psychology conference – be guided by any specialism you are developing as you undertake your clinical placements and your research, and target those conferences that will augment your expertise and put you in touch with the right people. This strategy can only stand in your favour when it comes time to seek employment. If someone at a conference shows interest in the work that you are doing, make sure to get in contact after the conference, indicating your desire to keep in touch about any future professional opportunities, and find a reason to drop them a line every once in a while.

Conferences can be expensive on top of an already-costly training, but the advantages for eventual employability can be worth it, and for the proactive and savvy trainee, conferencing can cost nothing whatsoever. Make sure you research and apply for any available bursaries from the conference organisers, your training institution, or your professional organisations. Again, when you volunteer on the conference committee or as a steward, you will almost always be able to attend free of charge.

Realise that there is a lull between training completion and registration – and plan for it

Counselling psychology training courses always specify how long the training takes – this could be between three and five years for the taught route. Understandably, then, you may assume that you will be qualified at the end of that time period, and fully ready to get out and get to work, HCPC registration card in hand. In the interest of managing expectations and helping you plan, however, I offer the following caveat. When counting down to registration, many (if not most) trainees do not realise that at the tail end of training there is often an enforced hiatus between the "end" – the turning in of the last coursework, or the submission of the thesis – and the point of qualification. This trainee explains more.

Third-year "plus" trainee counselling psychologist, awaiting viva:
It is quite common for counselling psychology trainees to be in a state of professional limbo, having finished training, but not yet being qualified due to having not yet completed doctoral research. Obviously it is preferable to not get into this position, and to be on top of the research side of the training concurrently with the clinical aspect; however, the reality is that this doesn't always happen. Amongst my own cohort, the majority of people, including me, have submitted their doctoral thesis a year or more after completing their professional training programmes.

I was fortunate enough to find some part-time paid work in a student counselling service, which helped me to keep working at the same time as carrying out research and writing up. I know other trainees who have found similar paid work before being qualified, e.g., as a therapist in IAPT (paid at Band 6 as therapist, rather than Band 7 as a psychologist). Such opportunities can arise out of being on placement within a service. Once they know your work and know you are competent, they might be prepared to offer you paid work. For this reason, it's useful to develop contacts when on placement. Make sure the head of service knows who you are, for example. I would advise trainees to consider a placement as a potential future job opportunity. Demonstrate all your professional skills! Offer to get involved in additional roles within the organisation, such as service evaluation and running workshops, rather than just going in to do the therapy hours.

I submitted my thesis some months ago and I am still waiting for my viva, a process that has taken several months and which is still ongoing. This may vary with different universities, but future trainees might want to be aware that even after submission, the whole process – including setting up the viva, having the viva, doing corrections, waiting for corrections to be approved, then through to HCPC registration – can in itself take several months.

Clearly, rather than succumbing to frustration or sitting home watching daytime television while you wait for your viva to happen or for the approval of your corrections, it is in your best interests to figure out what to do with your time in limbo. The trainee in the account above planned ahead and made connections during her training to enable her to get an interim job whilst awaiting registration, and this is a sound strategy. This is not all you can do, however.

All of the activities featured in the sections above – writing for publication, undertaking additional training, and conferencing – are productive and employability-enhancing activities that can productively fill your time between now and registration. If your viva has not yet occurred, or if you are waiting for the sign-off on your final corrections, be aware that you do not need to let your momentum drop – meet with your supervisor to start cutting down the work so that you can submit it for publication, keeping in mind that multiple distinct articles can be derived from one large doctoral thesis. Working with your research to distill the most salient arguments and significant findings into smaller journal articles can be excellent preparation for your viva, in which you will be required to present and defend your work clearly and succinctly. Conference, if you have not already – and if the last time you conferenced was when your work was in progress, it is probably time to conference again, in a different format this time, such as an individual paper. Are you ready, perhaps, to develop and offer a workshop or two, either on the conference circuit or off it? Finally, think about the areas in which you have developed a specialism, or a particular interest, over the course of your training. What can you do to develop those niches even further, so that you are that much more competitive when you are ready to apply for psychologist posts? Draw up a professional plan, isolating relative gaps in your competencies, or already-robust competencies that you can strengthen even further; identify ways of targeting those areas. The period between end of training and qualification need not be wasted time.

The importance of mentorship

Effective utilisation of one's own mentors is one of the factors differentiating a post-qualification success and a post-qualification fumble. Remember the graph in Figure 5.1 (Rosenberg, 2014), showing how your competence and proficiency can tail off after qualification if you do not have the proper support? Training is tough, and it can be hard to not be fully-fledged – as a consequence, many a newly-qualified counselling psychologist has been over-eager to put as much distance as possible between themselves and their erstwhile-trainee status. This has a potentially significant cost. In the novice professional stage – two to five years after qualification – trainees' competence and confidence can still be shaky, especially just after they fly the nest (Rønnestad & Skovholt, 2012). For many, finishing training means leaving behind the support of the cohort; the ready advice of tutors or Coordinating Supervisor; and the relative safety of training placements. Nevertheless, there are things that you can do to ensure that you have good continuity of support, sometimes with some of the same people who were supporting you before.

Mentorship for newly-qualified counselling psychologists can take several forms, and supervision is a given. All counselling psychologists, however senior, are expected to engage in regular supervision as long as they are in active practice. Psychologists who are more experienced may arrange peer supervision, but in the early years after qualification it is probably more beneficial and supportive to retain a more hierarchical supervisory relationship. For those who had training supervision exclusively within your clinical placements, you may not be able to access this once qualified, so you will need to do some shopping around, but think carefully about what you want from supervision at this stage before you rush into finding someone.

If you have already been using a supervisor independent of your clinical placement(s), you may keep seeing them through the transition from training through to early qualification, although you may also see this as an appropriate moment to make a change if your existing supervisor is not well placed to help you with work you are undertaking in a new job, or if you feel that a different type of supervisor might suit you best during the next phase of your professional development. If you are continuing with the same supervisor, have a supervision session where you explicitly discuss what you would like supervision to do for you now, and "re-contract".

Ongoing supervision is not just supportive, it helps ensure that you continue to practice ethically and safely, within the boundaries of your competence and for the benefit of your clients, as is required of all practitioner psychologists. Just being qualified is no guarantee that you will automatically do this, so your clinical supervision continues to be critical for reflective practice. Clinical supervisors, however, are not the only mentors that can be important in the post-qualification period. Particularly if you have not published or otherwise disseminated your work yet, keep meeting with your research supervisor(s) and/or other tutors who worked with you during training until you are ready to do so. A good working relationship with your trainers is one that can continue after qualification; you may undertake joint projects, or they may get you involved in the training from which you graduated, perhaps even as a visiting or guest lecturer.

Most of the academic tutors and supervisors providing professional training are likely to be, as so many counselling psychologists are, "portfolio professionals". To maintain their registration at least, and out of a sense of vocation and desire at most, they will do clinical work outside of the academic context. As such, some of them may be able to utilise their connections to help you into employment in the clinical sector, through writing references or perhaps more proactive assistance (if you have a strong relationship with them), and they can at least advise you, from a well-informed place, on your career. If the tutors or supervisors to whom you are closest are primarily academics, however, they are likely to undertake their clinical work on an independent-practice basis, and as a newly-qualified practitioner you might not be ready for this yet. (For more on this, see the next chapter.) If you are aiming to become an employee within the NHS or other settings (charities, educational settings, forensic settings, and so on), you may find that mentors within those settings will be more instrumental in supporting you in your fledgling post-qualification career.

Once you secure a post, while your manager or clinical supervisor on the job may serve as a mentor for you, it is probably better to seek guidance, support and advice from someone who is not a direct line manager or overseer/evaluator of your work. While in an ideal world you would be able to be transparent with your manager or a senior colleague about any uncertainties, difficulties or doubts you experience as you find your feet, you will probably feel more comfortable – and it is probably more circumspect – if you are most honest with someone who is not responsible for evaluating your performance. Consider approaching someone a few more years out from qualification, who has been through your stage of professional development relatively recently, or someone you connected with at a conference who works within your sector, or the sector within which you would like to work. Let them know that you are relatively newly-qualified and would really appreciate a discussion now and again with someone who could offer some advice, serve as a sounding board, or give a steer in a potentially useful direction. In my experience, most professionals – except perhaps the very busiest – are pleased to be able to offer their experience and their perspective.

The flip side to working with a mentor is *being* a mentor. As a novice professional, you may underestimate your ability to offer this. Imagine, however, the difference between someone who has just begun training and someone who has just completed it. Novice students – particularly a few months into training – are often convinced that they will never get a clinical placement, believe that they have made a horrible mistake in embarking on this journey, and wonder how they thought they could ever make it as counselling psychologists. Novice professionals have been there and done that, have gone through the stresses and the joys of training, and have accomplished all of the things that once seemed impossible. Acting as a mentor to people on the cohorts below you – whether informally with particular individuals you may have connected with, or formally through contributing to the course as a visiting or guest lecturer – not only helps others but serves you as well, by keeping you in touch with your trainers, paving the way for future employment at your own or other training institutions, and helping to solidify your growing sense of yourself as a qualified professional.

Working as a psychologist for the first time: securing employment

The shift from trainee to qualified counselling psychologist can feel rather strange. After years of informing each new client about your trainee status, and offering your services without charge (unless you were fortunate enough to have had paid placements), you may suffer from something like imposter syndrome when you begin applying for paying jobs, especially since your learning and developing in the post-qualification "novice professional" period remains on a reasonably steep curve. Nevertheless, securing your first post-qualification job will likely be at the forefront of your mind, and having the courage to sell yourself will be important.

Because counselling psychologists' backgrounds vary, the onus will be on you to be clear and assertive in selling yourself in the employment market. Put any insecurities aside and do a realistic yet confident audit of your professional competencies. Remember that training programmes approved by the BPS and HCPC need to show that their curricula will result in their graduates meeting dozens of standards of proficiency and competencies. If your training programme did not require you to map these out, now is the time to do it!

There are multiple formats for taking stock of your professional skills. One way is to make a log of precisely what you have done to meet each HCPC Standard of Proficiency (SOP). It is likely that some-where in your programme handbook(s) there is a mapping document of module learning outcomes or Documentary Evidence Units against the SOPs, and this is a good place to start. To make it more particular to you, think about specific essay titles, research topics, and presentations you have done over the course of your training, and what competencies these helped you show and specialisms these helped you develop. After you have completed that task, go on to consider all of the activities you undertook on clinical placements, and do not limit it to your face-to-face client sessions – after all, you probably performed a number of different tasks and roles in addition to psychotherapy sessions. Think too about all the workshops, talks, conferences, and other types of con-tinuing professional development you have done before, during, and after training. Do not forget about your previous, foundational psychol-ogy qualification (your BSc or your conversion diploma/MSc) – this is an important part of what qualifies you as a counselling psychologist, and make sure and include any other, specialist Master's work that you undertook before embarking on the doctorate. Page back through the syllabi and overall curricula for those qualifications, reacquaint yourself with the projects you did, and look at the specific learning outcomes for modules. Being specific about how you have met the standards should result in quite a large document, a comprehensive list from which you can pick and choose those elements that will be most relevant to particular advertised posts.

By mapping out the particulars of what you have done to meet not just counselling psychology-specific standards, but also the *generic* practitioner psychology standards (which constitute perhaps the majority of the SOPs document), you may find more confidence to apply for those job advertisements aimed at other types of practitioner psychologists. If you can do the job described, and can make a strong case for it, put yourself forward, keeping in mind that you may need a persuasive covering letter, a finely-honed CV that speaks directly to the post in question, and perhaps some personal contact with the organisation to maximise your chances of securing an interview in situations where counselling psychologists were not named in the advertisement.

Because the above method can generate such a large table of competencies, you may wish to organise your professional skills under a different kind of categorisation, for example, "Theoretical", "Clinical", "Research and measurement", "Teaching and training", "Leadership and management", "Supervision" and "Other" (you may think of some other specifics). The "Other" category can be more important than you imagine, as the accounts below show.

Case example 1: qualified counselling psychologist with a public relations background

This counselling psychologist describes using a range of skills beyond psychology to acquire and eventually keep a post in a sector in which she was relatively inexperienced. The post was supposed to last just a few months, but it morphed into a permanent post partly because of the skills she possessed from her previous career.

> *In an eating disorders job that I got through an agency, I noticed that one of the things that they really valued about me was my work experience. I had worked for public relations for ten years before retraining and had done budgets, worked with Excel, performed managerial duties, and so forth. The eating disorders service needed to do a lot of*

that, particularly as they were in the midst of trying to get professional accreditation through [a major UK eating disorders charity]. So, in addition to seeing clients, I helped with presentations and with getting recognition from that accrediting organisation. That really helped, in terms of how I got to stay on for so long!

Case example 2: qualified counselling psychologist with nursing background

In going for posts after qualification, this relatively newly-qualified counselling psychologist did not hesitate to use her nursing as well as her psychology skills to sell herself.

Having life experiences associated with a nursing background really helped. I worked in a field (renal transplant) where we had to communicate with patients about difficult and sensitive issues, things like non-adherence to treatment, transplant failure, cancer diagnoses, bereavement, and body image. Our patients were also from a broad range in terms of age, ethnicity, class, and so forth. I realised that there were lots of skills that I possessed that were transferable. If I could give one bit of advice regarding applying and interviewing, it would be to think outside the box as to where you may have got relevant skills, and don't be ashamed to really sell these, even they seem a bit tenuous. Let the interviewers make that judgement! I did this in terms of my former nursing role, and I didn't assume that people would know what psychology-relevant skills I might possess because I had been a nurse. Remember that each role is unique and what each person brings is unique, so explicitly state your case, as in "I did x job, which involved doing y, which demonstrates my awareness about and/or my ability to do z."

We live in a "competency culture". There is considerable overlap between different types of practitioner psychologists, in that they share a core group of generic proficiency standards, and your specific competencies will depend much on your particular training experiences, particularly your clinical placements. By the end of her training, one of the practitioners described above had accumulated considerable

CAMHS experience, making her highly competitive in that sector by the time she graduated, and her ability to work with that population was further enhanced by the CPD she undertook.

So, keep in mind that specific qualifications are important but not everything, and there may be many opportunities that are open to various types of practitioners, as long as those practitioners have the competencies outlined on the job description. Consider Improving Access to Psychological Therapies (IAPT) services within the NHS, for example. All types of practitioners – not just psychologists, but also psychotherapists, nurses, social workers, and other professionals – may work in IAPT, and are nearly always required to undergo extra training to try and ensure consistency in employees' ability to deliver services, whatever their existing qualifications. If you see a post that really grabs you, even if it specifies a particular type of qualification or registration that you do not have, ask for the person specification. Look closely at the essential and desirable criteria, scrutinise the job description, and weigh these up against the competency mapping that you have done. If you have the competencies that are needed, you may very well have a chance.

While the British Psychological Society's official website for jobs is www.psychapp.co.uk, and all NHS vacancies are advertised online at jobs.nhs.uk, you will also find jobs through agencies – enter "psychologist job agency" into a search engine to find out more and register with them. If you are interested in working within training/academia, www.jobs.ac.uk is the major jobs database within the UK. You can widen the net by maximising your credentials: if you do not have British Association for Counselling and Psychotherapy (BACP, www.bacp.co.uk) accredited status, or registration as a psychotherapist or counsellor with the United Kingdom Council for Psychotherapy (UKCP, www.ukcp.org.uk), visit their websites to see whether your training and experience qualifies you to for accreditation/registration.

In addition to keeping on top of particular job sites, plugging in the search terms that are relevant for you (for example, "psychologist psychotherapist counsellor jobs Manchester BPS UKCP") will quickly direct you to sites where jobs are posted; any time you find a new site that is useful to you, bookmark it and subscribe to be notified about new job postings, if the site offers that. You may also want to register with any one of the numerous agencies in the UK that specialise in placing practitioner psychologists, whether for permanent work or temporary/locum posts. The psychologist below described how agency work was perfect for her at a time when she wanted to expand her skill set somehow, but was not sure what sector would suit her.

Mid-career qualified counselling psychologist: *I gained one of my initial posts through connections made on placement, but I also have experience of getting an NHS job through an agency. Part of what attracted me to the agency was that, although I knew I wanted to stay in my specialist field [addictions], I also knew that I wanted to have some other experience so that I wasn't closing doors in the future. What kind of experience I wasn't sure, so an agency was a good way to explore that. Within weeks, the agency got me an interview for a three-month stint at an eating disorders service. Eating disorders had never interested me, but I thought, well, it's just three months, I could learn! I went for the interview, got the job, and three months turned into four or five years. For about two years that was through extensions of my agency contract, and then I applied for and got a permanent post, for which they had to advertise externally of course, but for which I was positioned very well.*

You may be wondering about another alternative: becoming self-employed through going into private practice straightaway upon qualification. This is a sufficiently contested issue to find a place in the next section, on challenges and issues within counselling psychology practice.

Challenges and issues within counselling psychology practice

Early qualification shares some challenges with training, and presents some of its own. There are also particular issues that are not just about being a novice professional, but which come with the professional territory, even for counselling psychologists who are quite experienced. Some of these, and potential ways of addressing them, have already been covered in the book: the potential for a drop-off in competencies without continuing support through supervision and continued learning, for example, and the competitiveness of the marketplace, in which one must sell oneself strategically through judicious and confident highlighting of one's competencies. This section covers a few more dilemmas or hurdles that a newly-qualified counselling psychologist may face, to include the question of private practice; the frustrations of encountering ignorance about or even prejudice towards the profession; and the trickiness of being a "portfolio professional".

Private practice as a newly-qualified counselling psychologist

As part of a developing portfolio career, or whilst waiting for the right employment to come along, independent practice can seem an attractive prospect. You have autonomy, flexibility, and a high degree of control over many aspects of your working life, but it has its challenges as well, as outlined below. Only you can judge whether you are at the right point to undertake it, and whether you have adequate professional support, both to ensure that you remain within the boundaries of your competence, and also to mitigate against the experience of isolation, particularly if you do not have any other working contexts.

If you take the plunge, even if you are only aiming to take on a few clients, remember that independent practice is a business. You may need to think about registering for self-employment tax, for example, and filing taxes as a self-employed person, which may come as a shock if you have always been a pay-as-you-earn (PAYE) employee. If you are processing client information on a computer, you may need to register with the Information Commissioner's Office (ICO). There may be implications for not just your professional liability insurance, but for your home, mortgage or renter's insurance if you are seeing clients from your primary residence. There are multiple issues to consider in setting up your own website, or when joining an online database of practitioners, and making decisions about your online presence is not as straightforward as it might seem. Suffice to say that to equip yourself adequately to start out in ethical, safe, business-aware independent practice, you should attend a course such as the one described by one of the psychologists in the case studies below; read published resources on the subject (e.g., Bor & Stokes, 2010); speak to any contacts you have who have experience in this area; and pore over the fine print in any tax regulations (using an accountant if you need to) and the terms and conditions of your insurance policies.

There are differing opinions on whether private practice straight out of qualification is a good idea. The scepticism of those in the "no" camp is understandable. Private practice, after all, is often referred to as "independent" practice. For newly-qualified people, at least for those who did not have existing qualifications or experience when they entered counselling psychology training, a choice to fly solo so soon after qualification may constitute more independence than they can handle, and they risk professional isolation and a drop-off in competence along the trajectory of Line C of Figure 5.1. The following accounts represent people who did decide to take the leap, two who did so virtually straightway upon qualification, and another who was comparatively cautious. These stories also give you a better flavour of what independent practice is like.

Newly-qualified counselling psychologist: *I was quite nervous about doing private practice straightaway. Nevertheless, I ended up doing it only three months after I qualified. I had worked quite independently in some of my placements, and people encouraged me to go for it, saying, "You might as well earn money for it, now that you're qualified." I also didn't yet have full-time work, so I had the capacity for it. It was very nerve-wracking to start with, because you never know who's going to walk through your door; there were some people from my course who had really challenging cases, and I was fortunate in that I didn't. I'm glad that I did it and got that experience and would probably encourage people to do it, as long as they have good supervision, good procedures, and good connections in place, such as established connections with GP practices or other people working in the area. It's probably particularly suited to people who have had experience of working quite independently in their placements. Now that I have a full-time post I've wound my private practice down, as it's just too much on top of my long hours! My dream is to do part-time work in an employment setting, but to also have the autonomy and flexibility of part-time private work, which I really like.*

Early-career counselling psychologist: *Private practice is something that I knew I always wanted to do, but I was unsure was whether or not I should get a few years' experience first, as a lot of people advised me – on the other hand, others said that the longer* *you leave it, the harder it is to make that jump, so I first went to an excellent British Psychological Society talk on setting up a private therapy service, and then I got myself set up working from home. I had looked into renting rooms, but for a number of reasons, I didn't think that was going to work for me, particularly because you usually have to make a commitment to regular sessions. I was concerned and didn't have the confidence at that stage; I was just starting out, I didn't know what clients or what hours I would have, and I didn't want to commit financially to doing it every week. I fixed up a room at home – made it quite minimalist – and started there. For referrals, I pursued a connection from my very first training placement in primary care, where the GP did NHS work but also had a private practice. That GP had asked me to get back in touch when I qualified, so that was my first port of call, and he immediately started referring me his private clients. It provided me with enough work that I didn't need to market myself to any other GPs – it got up to eight clients a week at one point.*

Mid-career counselling psychologist: *It took a few years to start to get into my private practice, because I didn't feel confident to go straight in after I finished training. My first post was a full-time teaching role in academia, and there was a lot going on. I did set up a consultancy early on, but it was a work in progress, and I didn't start advertising it straightaway because I just wanted to dedicate my time to my main job. When I did start independent practice, it was in a small conservatory type space that was slightly separate to my home, and I saw one or two clients a week. Thirteen years after qualification, my private practice is still fairly small in comparison to some, but you need to build and develop a private practice, and I've moved around quite a bit. Eventually I started renting a room in a place where there are a variety of other practitioners, and that has given me cross-referral relationships and has gotten my services more well-known.*

Selling yourself as an HCPC-registered counselling psychologist

As mentioned elsewhere in this book, all qualified counselling psychologists will share certain generic counselling psychology-specific proficiencies. Beyond these commonalities lies infinite variety, due to differences at both the training programme and the individual level. Compared to clinical psychology and counselling, it is also a newer profession, and one to which both laypeople and professionals may have had less exposure. If you are responding to a job advertisement that holds itself out as looking for a counselling psychologist (as the sole profession named, or as one specialisation listed amongst multiple), you are likely dealing with an organisation or department for whom counselling psychology is a known quantity. If you are responding to a listing that does not mention counselling psychology, or which only tentatively allows that counselling psychologists could possibly apply dependent upon experience, you will be on trickier footing. In such cases it is all very well to assume an optimistic attitude of *vive la différence*, but this will only pay off if potential employers understand the nature and extent of that *différence*, and they will likely wonder if your distinctiveness is of a type that adds value, or of a type that renders you insufficiently qualified to undertake the role. The examples below are examples of counselling psychologists who have encountered the latter situation, or who have experienced some level of personal tension between their professional identity and the context in which they work.

Qualified counselling psychologist: *Most of the counselling psychologists I know have had to explain several times to organisations, supervisors, clients and other people what counselling psychology is and what the difference is to clinical psychology, or we have had to differentiate between a "counselling psychologist" and a "counsellor". It feels a bit like being in a minority and having to fight to be heard and seen amongst other professionals.*

Qualified counselling psychologist: *I recently started a post in the NHS, having applied for several jobs. For many of these . . . they were also looking for other accreditation such as British Association for Behavioural & Cognitive Psychotherapies (BABCP). At one job interview, it was suggested to me that counselling psychology training did not necessarily give me the CBT expertise that I needed for the role. This was a bit depressing, given that in my opinion the counselling psychology training that I did goes above and beyond CBT training. Tension between the counselling psychology way and the IAPT way seems to vary from service to service. Once I ultimately started my* *job, I did feel strangely deskilled despite the depth and breadth of my training!*

Qualified counselling psychologist: *I wanted to be employed as a psychologist and not as a counsellor, and therefore I'd chosen NHS placements, which was helpful for securing NHS posts later on. However, there has been a considerable cost to this, and it has not always been easy to integrate my counselling psychology identity into my NHS work.*

Qualified counselling psychologist: *If you are going to work in the NHS, I think it is important to find a dialogue with clinical psychologists, as they will be your colleagues. Often in an NHS service there may be one counselling psychologist alongside two or three clinical psychologist colleagues. We offer different perspectives, but comparison and competition can feel negative – it's good to find points for collaboration.*

Nearly-qualified trainee counselling psychologist: *A newly-qualified friend was recently told that she did not have the right training for an NHS post – which, on paper, looked perfect for her – because she was a counselling and not a clinical psychologist. She did get an interview in the end, but sometimes it's a bit harder to "sell" yourself as a counselling psychologist. It's important that we promote what a counselling psychologist is, because no one else will.*

Virtually all of the counselling psychologists I have taught and supervised have had had little trouble gaining employment, many in their "first choice" sector. For those who do struggle to fight their corner, two points should be made. First, it helps to have a strong sense of your philosophy, values, and particular competencies. Second, a counselling psychologist can fit comfortably into nearly any working context that is consistent with his or her particular training history, clinical placement experience, and area(s) of research and scholarship, as the next chapter will further illustrate.

The ways in which you as an individual counselling psychologist can add value to a given post should be trumpeted in your CV, in your covering letters, and in your initial discussions and eventual interviews with potential employers. If it helps you or your would-be employers, look to the HCPC's *Standards of Proficiency* (2015) for help in positioning what you have to offer.

Being a portfolio professional

When speaking to counselling psychologists, you might notice that a particular phrase is used again and again: "portfolio professional" or "portfolio worker". When you are a full-time employee in one place, or if you are a sole trader focusing on providing one type of service, you will spend most or all of your time, and derive most (or all) of your income stream, from that activity. A portfolio professional or portfolio worker, on the other hand, "generates a multi-source income stream by working for diverse customers or doing a range of different activities" (Vermes, 2016, p. 619). I can give my own example: I work full-time as a Principal Lecturer and Head of Programmes for Counselling Psychology on a professional doctorate; I see between eight and ten clients and clinical supervisees per week; I provide research supervision and help with academic coursework on a consultancy basis; I undertake research and scholarship and do public speaking in that area; and I write book chapters and books such as this one.

Why do counselling psychologists so frequently construct their careers in a "portfolio worker" way? While there are no hard and fast statistics of which I am aware, nearly every counselling psychologist I know weaves together a tapestry of different roles and activities, and some – like myself – find themselves racing amongst multiple locations over the course of their working week. While I may be acquainted with a skewed sample or subset of counselling psychologists, the professionals I know generally find themselves not with too little work, but too much. Part of the problem seems to be that there is so much that they *can* do, and so much that seems interesting to them, that they find it difficult to edit their professional activities to a manageable workload. On the bright side, however, a portfolio worker can increase or decrease the number of things in their portfolio as their career evolves, or they can play with the relative percentages of time devoted to each activity as their current situation in life requires.

So, a counselling psychologist with multiple strings to their bow is rarely without some type of professional activity or income stream, even if they are, for example, taking some time out for family or other commitments. Despite the advantages of this, having multiple roles and responsibilities requires one to be a skilled juggler, and one practitioner describes her awareness of both sides of the coin.

Mid-career qualified counselling psychologist: *Because I have always done part private and part NHS, I am now in a very fortunate position. I have a particular specialism in the NHS, and now another practitioner who works within the same group as me wants to start a practice focused on that specialism, and has asked me join him as a partner. That business will be launching soon, and if it is as successful as we hope it will be, my aim is to eventually give up the NHS work for now. While I have always found the NHS to be very supportive and excellent when it comes to families, it has still been very challenging, because the amount of time you need off work can be tricky. That was one of the main reasons why I decided to go private initially, because I knew I could manage my time, and I wouldn't have to worry if I needed to be more flexible at any given point. The hardest thing I do, with all my work, is managing having two jobs and two young children.*

In this psychologist's situation, having had multiple things in her portfolio enabled her to respond more flexibly to life's demands than she would have been able to do had she only had one job – that is, had she been a sole trader, or had she possessed a full-time post with a single employer.

As has been mentioned so many times throughout this book, counselling psychologists in the UK can be found virtually anywhere that mental health services are offered. The final chapter in this book delves more richly and descriptively into what a career as a counselling psychologist can look like. Most of these in-depth case examples illustrate the portfolio nature of counselling psychology careers.

6 Career possibilities

While Chapter 2 of this book provided a broad overview of your job prospects within the field, the aim of this final chapter is to help you more vividly imagine the range of career possibilities in counselling psychology, through the medium of a number of case studies. These idiosyncratic portraits of professionals at work are not intended, of course, to be taken as templates – anyone who has read this far is aware that no such template really exists within counselling psychology – but they are intended to inspire you to follow wherever your preferences and aspirations lead you.

Throughout this book, you will have learned about the various specialisations counselling psychologists may pursue, and the diverse working contexts they might find themselves in. A more single-minded counselling psychologist may choose to specialise in just one aspect of professional activity, such as psychotherapeutic practice, service management, research, academia/training, supervision, or consultancy. Others combine one or more of these activities into a "portfolio career". In the pages that follow, you will get a sense of how no two portfolio careers in counselling psychology are alike!

Half NHS, half private: Hayley Melin, C.Psychol.

Large numbers of counselling psychologists are employed by the NHS but also incorporate independent practice into their working week. Hayley, a counselling psychologist who qualified within the last 10 years, has forged a successful working balance through a combination of NHS and private work.

I love the balance between NHS and private work. NHS work fits well with my values in terms of providing therapy for client groups who would otherwise not be able to access private therapy, I've always loved working with addictions, and I thoroughly enjoy the multidisciplinary team. (In private work you can have a multi-disciplinary team, but you have to build it yourself.) With private therapy, I specialise in addictions and eating disorders, but I get to work with everything, which provides variety and helps keeps me up to date.

My initial job in the NHS came about through connections from my first clinical placement. I had an early training placement in the addictions field, which I really enjoyed and where I had a very good relationship with my supervisor. Even after I qualified, when I was newly married and not wishing to apply for permanent jobs while expecting a baby, I decided to stay on placement with that supervisor. Even though I wasn't getting paid, my plan was to have the ends justify the means. One day the head of service approached me saying that he'd heard very good things and that he'd keep me in mind for future jobs in another service that he ran. Eventually that service called me, needing a psychologist for two days a week. I applied for the job and got it.

With private practice I started out by working from home. Because I was just starting out, I didn't want to commit financially to doing it every week. Again, connections I'd made during training served me well – the GP with whom I'd done one of my first training placements referred me his private clients. Eventually, a former student that I had supervised on placement asked if he could put my name forward for a newly-formed private-practice group, and that is where I now work. My luck or success in opportunities has always come about through knowing people, and training placements are really important for getting your name about, making connections, and building relationships. My advice is to always keep in contact, for your supervisors may one day be your colleagues!

Hayley describes appreciating the balance between NHS and private work, and this echoes the sentiments of many other CoPs I know. In harmony with the values of the field, she champions the ideal of socialised medicine: health care for all. The NHS as it functions currently, however, features some problematic characteristics outlined by Donati (2016): many services are high-pressure, high-stress working environments, significantly hindering reflective practice and limiting clinical autonomy. It is unsurprising, therefore, that many CoPs find the balance of NHS responsibilities and private work a more manageable combination of structure and flexibility, team working and independence, which also allows more time for the reflective practice, self-development, and self-care that is so important within the profession.

Developing your niche in the private setting: Jesse Tremblay, C.Psychol.

The NHS has taken responsibility for the health of the nation since its inception in 1948, but now there is deep concern in many quarters about its own continued health and wellbeing. Privatisation of UK health care is on the rise, and if the NHS still exists in a decade's time, it is nevertheless likely that private health care companies will be an additional major player on the scene, and a significant employer of counselling psychologists. The private sector is not a new phenomenon, of course, and for those with independent means and/or private health care insurance, psychological services in a private inpatient or outpatient environment have long been an option. In this case study, Jesse offers his perspective on working as a counselling psychologist in this type of setting.

> A few years before starting on my training, I bumped into a colleague from my undergraduate degree, who was a psychology assistant at a private hospital and helped me get an interview. Eventually this became my training placement for my counselling psychology programme, and it is where I still do most of my work today. I gained experience by shadowing colleagues under supervision and showed a keen and eager attitude, making myself known as reliable and indispensible.
>
> The best thing about the hospital is the range of professionals, from diverse training backgrounds, providing various treatment options. Clients can often have longer treatment, so we can be more integrative in approach and take time to test

formulations. As everyone's had different training, we can share ideas and sit in on each other's workshops, which fuels ideas and lively debate. To me this is real reflective practice, being challenged by colleagues who are also successful but who have completely different ideas regarding theory and approach.

If you work hard and have a strong can-do attitude you can make the right connections with consultants, who will remember you for future referrals. I have a nice mix of individual and group work, and I give weekly psycho-educational lectures and workshops to patients. Volunteering at open evenings, to help the hospital pitch treatment programmes and personal specialties to large groups of GPs and psychiatrists, is a good way to get known and to get referrals.

At this point in my career, having initially worked under a contract to establish myself, I am now a sessional psychologist consulting independently for the hospital. This has financial benefits and gives enormous flexibility to my work life – for example, I frequently work hard for a couple of days then take the rest of the week off, or do morning or evening clinics here and there, allowing me to do other things to keep my personal balance. Sessional work is really like running your own private business, so you need to make good connections to get referrals. In my private practice so far I've relied on word of mouth and a good reputation rather than advertising, and I have a steady stream of referrals from large private organisations and established consultants.

The longer I have been practising, the more I have taken note of the importance of holistic wellbeing. I'm now doing a Master's looking into the effects of nutrition and fitness on everything: hormone changes, weight regulation, energy levels, and mood. I'm now designing my own weekly workshop around this, to add to the already-extensive programme offered to inpatients and day patients. If you have a passion and push yourself, there is great scope to develop personal interests within the private sector.

Forging your own path and developing specialisms may be possible within NHS work, but it may be easier to achieve this in the private sector. Through working hard, nurturing professional relationships, and following his passions, Jesse has developed his career in a way that he has a marketable niche specialism and a steady flow of referrals.

The more established he has become, the more flexibility he has had to pursue the best balance between work and the rest of his life, and private clinic work represents a percentage of his income too. In his private clinics he is registered with many private health insurance companies, which can be extremely important for private practitioners. It is important to be aware, however, that certain providers may require you to be many years post-qualification (as many as seven) before you can join their list.

Full-time, independent school: a "novice professional" counselling psychologist

Not everyone, of course, aspires to a career in either an NHS or private clinical setting. Even though counselling psychology training focuses on preparing graduates to work with an adult population within clinical settings, the right balance of placement experiences, supervisory support, and CPD can open a variety of doors. This psychologist used her placement experiences from training as a springboard onto a different path – counselling within the independent-school sector. (She felt most comfortable staying anonymous while sharing her experiences, which partially relate to her current employment.)

> A lot of my peers were quite keen to work in the NHS, but I was looking for something different. At the start of my training I wanted to work in schools, so I began my training with a school placement. My programme limited how many "child hours" I could count towards accreditation, however, so after my first year I shifted to adult work. While still pre-qualification and awaiting confirmation of my thesis corrections, I got my first paid job with my original training placement, as an assistant school project manager. While being more a managerial than a clinical role, it taught me how a service worked in a school.
>
> My first post-qualification job was at an independent preparatory school, where my title was school counsellor. I did one-to-one work as well as personal, social, health and economic education (PSHE) lessons. I hadn't done teaching before. I had to deal with school dynamics and communications with parents, I was relatively

inexperienced, and as I worked autonomously I was relatively isolated. It was also only part-time, so I found a concurrent job in another independent school. In both places CPD wasn't provided, so I had to take initiative to develop my practice – for example, I undertook an "Understanding Adolescents" course and did other reading and research to fill gaps in my knowledge.

Recently I became aware of a full-time post being offered at another independent school. I wasn't even looking for a job – my partner is a teacher and saw the post advertised. Because they specified clinical psychology, I was unsure about applying, but it fit with my experience and my supervisor encouraged me. During my interview, the panel – including a clinical psychologist – asked me why I'd chosen to study counselling instead of clinical psychology. I replied that I was keen to work in a variety of environments, including GP surgeries and schools, and that counselling psychology training had enabled me to do that, and I really showed my confidence in, and my valuing of, counselling psychology. They offered me the post. It's been challenging shifting to full-time, running a service, having more responsibility, and managing a large caseload, but on the other hand, working alongside other professionals – school doctors and psychiatrists – means I'm less isolated than in my previous roles. I have more of a sense of belonging, and a sense that people really understand my role and purpose.

I would advise any newly-qualified counselling psychologist to take time to think about what you want to do. What are you passionate about? What have you enjoyed in your training? Realise that it's possible to work in settings outside of the NHS. You may end up going down a route where you're not in a team, or where you have less support in your role, but you can be fine and can develop as long as you get good supervision and support.

This psychologist's case study is another illustration of how clinical placement choices can pave the way for a future career, but it is also an instance of an appropriately experienced counselling psychologist successfully arguing her suitability for a particular role, even though the people advertising that post were expecting to hire another type of psychology professional. In telling her story, this novice professional expressed a certain self-consciousness about her career trajectory thus far; to an extent, she said, she developed her specialisation through responding to opportunity, rather than through proceeding with deliberate intent. This is not, however, unusual for someone in this phase of career.

Entrepreneur and Registrar for the QCoP: Dr Victoria Galbraith, C.Psychol.

More seasoned professionals tend to have a more developed sense of themselves personally and professionally and a certain level of confidence, from which vantage point they can more deliberately consider and choose their next career steps. One of the developmental tasks of the experienced-professional phase is "for the [practitioner] to create a work role which is experienced as highly congruent with the practitioner's coherent professional self" (Rønnestad & Skovholt, 2012, p. 98). Victoria's story illustrates how one experienced professional took the road less travelled, in service of finding a greater level of personal and professional congruence.

Sixteen years ago, newly-qualified, I could have taken a post at what had been my clinical placement; instead, I went for a university post. I built my confidence in teaching counselling psychology at undergraduate and postgraduate levels, and in time was promoted to Senior Lecturer, whilst also maintaining a small private practice. I gained experience in developing curriculums and preparing programmes for validation at another academic post, and ultimately I took a leading role in completely rewriting my counselling psychology programme, and taking it through revalidation and BPS accreditation.

I was delighted that I'd designed a good programme that received lots of commendations, and I stayed on in my post for about a year afterwards, but I began to feel that I'd done everything I'd aspired to do in that area. I wanted to focus more on wellbeing, to use my counselling psychology skills and way of being in a different way, and to apply understanding from psychological theory in a different context. I was particularly interested in taking therapy outdoors and had a personal as well as a professional motivation for this – I realised that since moving inland from Wales, I missed being near the coast. I also wanted to develop something that was for everybody, not just for people that were suffering from distress, so that anyone could learn more about themselves, have some time out, and use the sea as a way of facilitating that. I resigned from my university post, took a nature connectedness course to understand more about engaging with nature safely, and eventually launched Seacotherapy, which involves retreats incorporating coastal activities and therapeutic practices, such as mindfulness, near water.

In addition to running Seacotherapy, I recently became the Registrar for the Qualification in Counselling Psychology (QCoP). Although it's a learning curve because I wasn't particularly familiar with the Qualification, in other ways it was a natural progression because I'd been on the BPS training committee, I'd been a programme leader, and I understood professional training through doing accreditations and external examinations. I've also become involved with writing and editing. An editor of *The Handbook of Counselling Psychology* approached me about doing a chapter, but then asked if I'd like to co-edit. I jumped at the chance to be involved with the core text for the profession, a book I'd used in my own training and beyond. That's opened more doors, and I successfully made a proposal for an edited book of my own. There isn't a text like it available yet, so it's fresh, new and a great opportunity.

I would advise other counselling psychologists to be creative. Know what's required in terms of competencies, standards of proficiency and ethics, but within that, think about how counselling psychology can be developed and how you can take the profession into other domains. I think there's so much scope for that!

Victoria has come to her current combination of work activities after many shifts and changes; she has reflected on not just what she wants for herself, but what she wants counselling psychology to do for others. As her career has evolved, so has her way of combining applied practice and academic work.

Lecturer, practitioner, and passionate researcher: Dr Edith Steffen, C.Psychol.

As the last example and this one shows, academia and/or training represents a significant employment opportunity for counselling psychologists, and is an excellent way of promoting ongoing developing and learning for the teacher as well as the pupil. You can be involved in lecturing on a variety of levels, from giving workshops or being an occasional visiting lecturer to being a full-time permanent faculty member. Because ongoing registration and chartership requires counselling psychologists to maintain clinical practice, the academic/clinician juggling act will be familiar to most counselling psychologists who are involved in teaching and training others, and for those professionals who want to focus more deeply on scholarship and research, it can be challenging to include everything one desires in one's portfolio of valued activities. Edith's case study illustrates an early-career counselling psychologist attempting to follow her passions and to get the balance right.

My dream had been to be part academic and part practitioner, and I used to work 2.5 days at a university and 2.5 days in a community mental health service, but I am now a full-time lecturer on a counselling psychology programme, with a small private practice. I changed to a full-time post to enable me to do research, for I found it very difficult, if not impossible, to do research as a part-time academic. I think it is regrettable that research is not generally an *integral* aspect of the work of a counselling psychologist.

For me, the joy of being a counselling psychologist is that I love the learning: there is always so much to learn, whether you work in practice or in academia. It is such a rich working life, and to me it is not a job but living my passion, living my dream. I do find it a lot easier to be an academic than a practitioner, and I am not sure whether that just says a lot about me or whether that says something about the role of a therapist, which is never easy. While working with clients gives me a lot more satisfaction on a day-to-day level than a day's academic workload, on a grander scale being an academic fulfils me more, as it combines a greater range of what matters to me. That includes engaging in scholarly debates while still growing as a therapist, working with texts as well as supporting students in their learning, and communicating with a vast number of people, as well as spending many quiet hours by myself, just reading and writing. The downside of academic life may be the administrative side of things; many hours of the working day are spent responding to emails, filling in forms, ticking boxes and following procedures. The perfect job for me would therefore be one where I could be a researcher, a therapist and a lecturer but not have any administrative duties! Having said that, administration in academia is a bit like housework in your home. If everyone does a little bit of it, it doesn't get too daunting. Sometimes it feels quite nice to be able to get a job done that helps the whole team.

Edith's account of trying to be both an academic and a practitioner, while also undertaking research, has strong personal resonance, for I too attempt to stay involved across this range of professional activities. Research has enriched and enlivened my own practice and professional career, not to mention enhanced my employability, and I would argue that doing research that really matters and that benefits both individual clients and society at large is an important way of realising the humanistic ethos at the heart of counselling psychology, as well as promoting lifelong learning and development.

Counselling psychologist specialising in pain, Ministry of Defence: Dr Ellen Murphy, C.Psychol

While the case studies thus far primarily involve working contexts that you might have expected or thought of – clinical practice, academia, research, private work – Ellen, the psychologist in our final example, found her "dream job" working in a less common setting.

I'd always been drawn to working with trauma, and while waiting for my doctorate to be ratified, I saw a job advertised by the Ministry of Defence (MoD) for a counselling or clinical psychologist. I phoned for clarity about the role, and they were looking for a psychologist who could think in a psychological way about pain and who could develop and implement a new programme. I'd worked in end-of-life care and dealt with pain issues there, and I thought, well, I can do that! At interview they were very interested in the way I talked about pain and psychology, particularly my relational approach – it was just what they were looking for. I became the first psychologist specialising in pain within the MoD, and was able to come in as a Lieutenant Colonel at Band 8a, which was fantastic for a newly-qualified psychologist.

Not only was the job role brand new, but I was also newly-qualified, in an organisation that was new to me, working with a population I didn't know, within an unfamiliar three-week model of therapy. The patients are admitted to my rehabilitation centre for three weeks, during which time I try and optimise their rehab outcome. All those layers of novelty made it a baptism by fire, and I had to rely on my flexibility and creativity. I also did a lot of post-qualification reading and CPD to bring myself up to speed, and I'm now trained in EMDR Levels 1, 2 and 3, Compassion-Focused Therapy (CFT), Acceptance & Commitment Therapy (ACT), trauma-focused CBT, and hypnosis for pain.

I think I became fully rounded as a psychologist in this role; this is where I feel like my identity and competence has grown and settled. Now I forge links with other pain management services, consult with the mental health centres that are linked to barracks all over the country, and go to international conferences. I also do a lot of in-service training and CPD, teaching people about psychological responses to pain. I'm embedded within the whole rehabilitation centre, working across five teams and alongside many other types professionals: occupational therapists, physiotherapists, consultants, medical doctors, recreational therapists, social workers, community psychiatric nurses, neuropsychologists, and a mild traumatic brain injury psychologist.

As a counselling psychologist I work quite differently to many of my professional colleagues. The demographic I work with responds very well to a relational, intuitive, creative, flexible, kind of working. I build a therapeutic alliance with clients very quickly, and I think that comes from my training. In addition, because I'm existentially orientated, my formulations really promote understanding about why the patient is experiencing these difficulties at this time, and that's highly valued within the team.

My whole training journey provided me with the backbone to put myself in situations that are challenging and anxiety-provoking. I've now stood up in front of 400 staff and presented – something I never would have wanted to do a few years ago – and I've got the confidence now to do so many other things. I have the title "Pain

Psychologist", but I always let people know that I'm a counselling psychologist with a specialism in pain. I'm proud of that identity, and I want to protect it.

The diversity in these six case studies is just the tip of the iceberg, a mere hint of the even greater variety that exists beyond the pages of this book. The possibilities for the creative, entrepreneurial counselling psychologist are vast indeed, limited only by the individual professional's imagination. As the Microsoft advertising slogan of some two decades ago asked: "Where do you want to go today?"

Counselling psychology career possibilities in other countries

We live in an increasingly mobile society, and for some UK-trained CoPs, the answer to "Where do you want to go today?" might be "Someplace else!" Life has many twists and turns, and one day you may find yourself wondering if you can take your counselling psychology career and hit the road with it.

In 2002 the profession of counselling psychology gained division status with the International Association of Applied Psychology (IAAP), an organisation that exists to "promote the science and practice of applied psychology and to facilitate interaction and communication about applied psychology around the world" (www.iaapsy.org). This does not mean, however, that universal qualification exists, and the field is constituted differently in various spots around the globe. In some countries the field of counselling psychology is regulated and the title of "counselling psychologist" legally protected; in others, psychology is regulated but "counselling psychology" not formally recognised (James, 2016; Orlans & van Scoyoc, 2009).

Because recognised titles, professional standards, and professional trainings can differ significantly, a counselling psychologist becoming accredited, registered and/or licensed across different countries can range from tricky at best to impossible at worst.

The bottom line is that you should never assume that doing a UK counselling psychology training programme would result in your being able to practice as a counselling psychologist elsewhere. If you have plans or aspirations to live and work abroad, always *thoroughly* consult the relevant professional regulatory departments in the country to which you plan on emigrating. In some cases, even if you do not automatically qualify to trade as a counselling psychologist, you may still find yourself able to gain another type of licensure or registration that enables you to practice, for example, the LCPC (Licensed Clinical Professional Counsellor) qualification in some areas of the United States.

James (2016) discusses numerous organisations that are endeavouring to make transfer of qualifications easier. For example, the European Federation of Psychologists Association is working towards qualification across European countries, but at the time of writing, only clinical/ health psychology, work/organisational psychology, and educational psychology are explicitly identified as being eligible for the EuroPsy register. While moving abroad does not mean that you will never (re) gain your ability to practice as a counselling psychologist or to call yourself by that title, it certainly means that you will have a number of hoops through which to jump. Look before you leap!

Final word

If this book has done its job well, you will now have a richer sense of the diverse profession of counselling psychology. Perhaps your curiosity has been piqued, and you would like to explore further. Maybe you have even been sufficiently inspired to take the next steps, in hopes of becoming a trainee and eventually joining our ranks as a colleague. In either case, the Appendix lists organisations and websites that will help you find out more. If you have an aptitude and passion for psychological practice, if you are committed to doing work that benefits both individuals and the wider world, and if you intend to keep learning and developing for the duration of your career, we hope that we will be hearing much more from you. Welcome to the field.

Appendix

Useful information

Acronyms and websites

AEC   Accreditation of Existing Competence. Some training programmes, and the Qualification in Counselling Psychology, will accept AEC for credit if you have had significant prior learning, training or experience that gives you a particular competency.

BA   Bachelor of Arts, a Level-6 qualification in the United Kingdom.

BABCP   British Association for Behavioural & Cognitive Psychotherapies, a voluntary registering body for practitioners specialised and qualified in cognitive behavioural therapy. See www.babcp.com

BACP   British Association for Counselling and Psychotherapy, a voluntary registering body for qualified counsellors and psychotherapists in the United Kingdom. See www.bacp.co.uk

BPS   British Psychological Society. The learned society and professional body for psychologists in the United Kingdom. See www.bps.org.uk

BSc   Bachelor of Science, a Level-6 qualification in the United Kingdom.

CAMHS   An acronym for Child & Adolescent Mental Health Services, historically a specialist department within the National Health Service.

CBT   Cognitive-behavioural therapy, one modality of talking therapy and the primary modality offered

	by Improving Access to Psychological Therapies (IAPT) services in the UK.
CoP	A common acronym for counselling psychology.
CPD	Continuing professional development, a requirement of all practitioner psychologists post qualification.
C.Psychol.	The designation for Chartered Psychologist, indicating that a psychologist is chartered by the British Psychological Society.
CS	Coordinating Supervisor. The CS oversees training for a candidate on the QCoP or Independent Route.
DBS	Disclosure and Barring Service. A DBS check picks up any criminal history and is undertaken to ensure a practitioner is safe to work with clients, particularly clients in vulnerable populations.
DCoP	The Division of Counselling Psychology. See www.bps.org.uk/dcop
DPsych, DCounsPsy, DCPsych, PsychD	Abbreviations for a practitioner doctorate in counselling psychology, all of which refer to the same type of degree.
DSM-5	Diagnostic and Statistical Manual of Mental Disorders, a diagnostic taxonomy of psychological disorders, now in its 5th edition.
EAP	Employee Assistance Programme, schemes that provide emotional, psychological, and general wellbeing support to employees.
GBC	Graduate Basis for Chartership, the baseline requirement for postgraduate study in psychology in the UK.
GBR	Graduate Basis for Registration, a now-out-of-use designation that was the equivalent of GBC when the BPS was still the registering body for psychologists.
HCPC	The Health and Care Professions Council. The body which has been the statutory regulating organisation for all practitioner psychologists since 2009. Only HCPC-registered practitioner psychologists may use protected titles such as "Counselling Psychologist". See www.hcpc-uk.co.uk

IAAP	International Association of Applied Psychology, the oldest international association of psychologists, which aims to "promote the science and practice of applied psychology and to facilitate interaction and communication about applied psychology around the world". See www.iaapsy.org
IAPT	Improving Access to Psychological Therapies, an English programme to improve access to talking therapies on the National Health Service. See www.iapt.nhs.uk
ICD-10	The International Classification of Diseases, a diagnostic taxonomy of disease and disorder, to include psychological difficulties; it is now in its 10th edition.
LD	An acronym for learning difficulties. Clients with learning difficulties have historically been treated within specialist LD services within the National Health Service.
MA	Master of Arts degree, classified as a Level-7 degree in the United Kingdom, usually involving a Master's thesis but not necessarily a piece of research.
MBPsS	Designation for a Graduate Member of the British Psychological Society, which confers Graduate Basis for Chartership.
MSc	Master of Science degree, classified as a Level-7 degree in the United Kingdom, usually involving a research-orientated Master's thesis.
NARIC	The designated national agency in the UK for recognition and comparision of international qualifications and skills. See www.naric.org.uk
NHS	National Health Service, the system of socialised health care that has provided free health care at point of use for every resident of the United Kingdom since its inception in 1948. See www.nhs.uk
NHS Employers	Information about current pay scales for psychologists can be found on http://www.nhsemployers.org
NVQ	National Vocational Qualification.
PGCert	Postgraduate Certificate.
PGDip	Postgraduate Diploma.

PWP	Psychological Wellbeing Practitioner, a role within Improving Access to Psychological Therapies that is accessible to psychology graduates. See www.bps.org.uk/pwp
QAA	The Quality Assurance Agency for Higher Education. An independent body that monitors and advises on standards and quality in UK education. The QAA sets benchmarks for study in various subjects, such as psychology, as well as qualification descriptors for various levels of educational degrees. See www.qaa.ac.uk
QCoP	The Qualification in Counselling Psychology, also known as the Independent Route, a BPS qualification route to becoming a counselling psychologist. The QCoP is an alternative to the doctoral-level course route. See www.bps.org.uk/careers-education-training/society-qualifications/counselling-psychology/counselling-psychology
RQF	Regulated Qualifications Framework. The RQF in the UK is a single system for cataloguing qualifications by level and size.
SETs	Standards of Education and Training, the standards that the Health and Care Professions Council sets for training practitioner psychologists and other professionals that the HCPC regulates. See www.hcpc-uk.co.uk
SOPs	Standards of Proficiency, the standards that practitioner psychologists must meet in order to qualify as registered with the HCPC. See www.hcpc-uk.co.uk
UKCP	United Kingdom Council for Psychotherapy, a voluntary registering body for qualified psychotherapists in the United Kingdom. See www.ukcp.org.uk

Additional electronic resources

- @dcopuk: Twitter handle for the Division of Counselling Psychology.
- Counselling Psychologists UK: closed Facebook group for UK CoPs and CoPs in training.

- Qualifications Office of the BPS: www.bps.org.uk/careers-education-training/society-qualifications/qualifications-teamcontact-us/qualifications-office

- London Counselling Psychologists: a consultancy that supports aspiring and existing counselling psychology trainees. See www.londoncounsellingpsychologists.co.uk

- BPS jobs website: see www.psychapp.co.uk

- Jobs.ac.uk: The primary jobs website for academics in the UK. See www.jobs.ac.uk

Bibliography

Bor, R. & Stokes, A. (2010). *Setting up in independent practice: A handbook for counsellors, therapists and psychologists.* London: Palgrave Macmillan.

Bor, R. & Watts, M. (2016). *The trainee handbook* (4th ed.). London: SAGE Publications Ltd.

British Psychological Society (2015). *Standards for the accreditation of doctoral programmes in counselling psychology.* Available on: http://bps.org.uk/system/files/Public%20files/PaCT/counselling_accreditation_2015_web.pdf. Accessed 12 March 2016.

British Psychological Society (2016). Careers – Counselling Psychology. Available on: http://careers.bps.org.uk/area/counselling. Accessed 12 March 2016.

Davey, G. (Ed.) (2013). *Applied Psychology* [Six Supplementary Chapters]. Available on: http://bcs.wiley.com/he-bcs/Books?action=resource&bcsId=6483&itemId=1444331213&resourceId=29364. Accessed 19 March 2016.

Donati, M. (2016). Becoming a reflective practitioner. In B. Douglas, R. Woolfe, S. Strawbridge, E. Kasket & V. Galbraith (Eds.), *The handbook of counselling psychology* (4th ed.) (pp. 55–73). London: SAGE Publications Ltd.

Douglas, B., Woolfe, R., Strawbridge, S., Kasket E., & Galbraith, V. (2016). *The handbook of counselling psychology* (4th ed.). London: SAGE Publications Ltd.

Galbraith, V. (2016). Engaging with academia and training programmes. In B. Douglas, R. Woolfe, S. Strawbridge, E. Kasket & V. Galbraith (Eds.), *The handbook of counselling psychology* (4th ed.) (pp. 74–92). London: SAGE Publications Ltd.

Gkouskos, S. (2016). Becoming a trainee. In B. Douglas, R. Woolfe, S. Strawbridge, E. Kasket & V. Galbraith (Eds.), *The handbook of counselling psychology* (4th ed.) (pp. 600–615). London: SAGE Publications Ltd.

Hanley, T., Cutts, L., Gordon, R., & Scott, A. (2013). A research-informed approach to counselling psychology [Supplementary Chapter, Student Companion Site]. In G. Davey (Ed.), *Applied psychology.* Available on: http://bcs.wiley.com/he-bcs/Books?action=mininav&bcsId=6483&itemId=1444331213&assetId=297218&resourceId=29364&newwindow=true. Accessed 13 March 2016.

Hanley, T., Steffen, E., & O'Hara, D. (2016). Research: From consumer to producer. In B. Douglas, R. Woolfe, S. Strawbridge, E. Kasket & V. Galbraith (Eds.), *The handbook of counselling psychology* (4th ed.) (pp. 530–546). London: SAGE Publications Ltd.

Health and Care Professions Council (2012). *Standards of conduct, performance, and ethics.* Available on: http://www.hcpc-uk.org.uk/assets/documents/100 03B6EStandardsofconduct,performanceandethics.pdf. Accessed 22 May 2016.

Health and Care Professions Council (2015). *Standards of proficiency: Practitioner psychologists.* Available on: http://hpc-uk.org/assets/documents/ 10002963sop_practitioner_psychologists.pdf. Accessed 12 March 2016.

Health and Care Professions Council (n.d.). *International application for registration.* Available on: http://www.hcpc-uk.org/assets/documents/ 10003B02HCPC-Application-pack-International.pdf. Accessed on 12 March 2016.

Henton, I. (2016). Engaging with research. In B. Douglas, R. Woolfe, S. Strawbridge, E. Kasket & V. Galbraith (Eds.), *The handbook of counselling psychology* (4th ed.) (pp. 132–148). London: SAGE Publications Ltd.

Henton, I., & Kasket, E. (2017). Research in counselling psychology. In V. Galbraith (Ed.), *Counselling psychology.* London: Routledge.

Hitchings, P. (2016). Becoming a supervisee. In B. Douglas, R. Woolfe, S. Strawbridge, E. Kasket & V. Galbraith (Eds.), *The handbook of counselling psychology* (4th ed.) (pp. 112–131). London: SAGE Publications Ltd.

Hitchings, P. and Ornellas, J. (2011). Preparing for a job after professional registration. In R. Bor & M. Watts, *The trainee handbook* (3rd ed.) (pp. 356–369). London: SAGE Publications Ltd.

James, P. (2016). Counselling psychology and its international dimensions. In B. Douglas, R. Woolfe, S. Strawbridge, E. Kasket & V. Galbraith (Eds.), *The handbook of counselling psychology* (4th ed.) (pp. 399–414). London: SAGE Publications Ltd.

Kasket, E. (2013). The counselling psychologist researcher [Supplementary Chapter, Student Companion Site]. In G. Davey (Ed.), *Applied psychology.* Available on: http://bcs.wiley.com/he-bcs/Books?action=mininav&bcsId =6483&itemId=1444331213&assetId=297219&resourceId=29364&new window=true. Accessed 13 March 2016.

Kasket, E. (2016a). Carrying out research. In B. Douglas, R. Woolfe, S. Strawbridge, E. Kasket & V. Galbraith (Eds.), *The handbook of counselling psychology* (4th ed.) (pp. 530–546). London: SAGE Publications Ltd.

Kasket, E. (2016b). Researching across the career span. In B. Douglas, R. Woolfe, S. Strawbridge, E. Kasket & V. Galbraith (Eds.), *The handbook of counselling psychology* (4th ed.) (pp. 228–243). London: SAGE Publications Ltd.

Kasket, E. (2016c). Preparing for a job after professional registration. In R. Bor & M. Watts (Eds.), *The trainee handbook* (4th ed.) (pp. 387–400). London: SAGE Publications Ltd.

Kasket, E. & Gil-Rodriguez, E. (2012). The identity crisis in trainee counselling psychology research. *Counselling Psychology Review, 26*(4), pp. 20–30.

Lane, D., & Corrie, S. (2006). Counselling psychology: Its influences and future. *Counselling Psychology Review, 21*(1), pp. 12–24.

Lawrence, J. (2016). Entering clinical placements. In B. Douglas, R. Woolfe, S. Strawbridge, E. Kasket & V. Galbraith (Eds.), *The handbook of counselling psychology* (4th ed.) (pp. 93–111). London: SAGE Publications Ltd.

Orlans, V., & van Scoyoc, S. (2009). *A short introduction to counselling psychology.* London: SAGE Publications Ltd.

Quality Assurance Agency (2010). *Subject benchmark statement: Psychology.* Available on: http://qaa.ac.uk/en/Publications/Documents/Subject-benchmark-statement-Psychology.pdf. Accessed 12 March 2015.

Rafalin, D. (2010). Counselling psychology and research: Revisiting the relationship in light of our 'mission'. In M. Milton (Ed.), *Therapy and beyond: Counselling psychology contributions to therapeutic and social issues* (pp. 41–56). Chichester, UK: John Wiley & Sons.

Robson, C. & McCartain, K. (2015). *Real world research.* Chichester, UK: John Wiley & Sons.

Rønnestad, M. H., & Skovholt, T. (2012). *The developing practitioner: Growth and stagnation of therapists and counselors.* New York: Routledge.

Rosenberg, M. (2014). Why support after training is important [Internet Article]. Available on: http://learningsolutionsmag.com/articles/1348/marc-my-words-the-training-to-competence-myth. Accessed 27 February 2017.

Schön, D. A. (1983). *The reflective practitioner: How professionals think in action.* New York: Basic Books.

Thomson, P., & Kamler, B. (2012). *Writing for peer reviewed journals: Strategies for getting published.* London: Routledge.

Vermes, C. (2016). Becoming an entrepreneur-practitioner. In B. Douglas, R. Woolfe, S. Strawbridge, E. Kasket & V. Galbraith (Eds.), *The handbook of counselling psychology* (4th ed.) (pp. 616–639). London: SAGE Publications Ltd.

Vossler, A., & Moller, N. (2015). *The counselling and psychotherapy research handbook.* London: SAGE Publications Ltd.

Yalom, I. (2003). *The gift of therapy: An open letter to a new generation of therapists and their patients: Reflections on being a therapist.* London: Piatkus.

Index